The Cure Is in the Kitchen

. . . or perhaps, the garden. In this comprehensive compendium of simple, easily accessible natural remedies for the home treatment of minor ailments and injuries, a leading English herbalist introduces us to the amazing world of medicinal herbs, vegetables and fruits and teaches us how to turn them into healing teas, oils and compresses to ease 50 common discomforts from colds and cuts to the pain of arthritis and gastric distress.

About the Author

Penelope Ody majored in chemistry at Bristol University in England. Later she studied herbal medicine at the School of Phytotherapy in Sussex and traditional Chinese medicine at the College of Traditional Chinese Medicine in Guangzhou. She is a member of the National Institute of Medical Herbalists, England's leading professional body for practicing herbalists. Ody's previous herb books include *The Complete Medicinal Herbal, Home Herbal, Handbook of Over-the-Counter Herbal Medicines, Pocket Medicinal Herbs* and *101 Natural Remedies.*

Her herb garden in Buckinghamshire, where she practiced as a consultant medical herbalist for 10 years, has been featured on BBC Television. She now lives in Hampshire and continues to contribute to a number of publications worldwide and lecture on herbal medicine throughout the world.

Keats Publishing, Inc. ▪ New Canaan, C

A KEATS GOOD HERB GUIDE

MEDICINE
FOR THE
21 CENTURY

HERBS FOR FIRST AID

*Simple home remedies for minor
ailments and injuries from coughs
and colds to cuts and bruises*

Penelope Ody

Keats Publishing, Inc. ❦ New Canaan, Connecticut

For John Clive
with love

HERBS FOR FIRST AID

Copyright © 1997 by Penelope Ody

Library of Congress Cataloging-in-Publication Data

Ody, Penelope.
    Herbs for first aid / Penelope Ody.
      p.   cm.
    Includes bibliographical references and index.
    ISBN 0-87983-825-6
    1. Herbs—Therapeutic use.   2. First aid in illness and injury.
  I. Title.
RM666.H330382 1997
615'.321—dc21
                                    97-27554
                                      CIP

Printed in the United States of America

Keats Good Herb Guides are published by
Keats Publishing, Inc.
27 Pine Street (Box 876)
New Canaan, Connecticut 06840-0876

Keats Publishing website address: www.Keats.com

99 98 97   6 5 4 3 2 1

Contents

Introduction

"First aid" to most people conjures an image of splints and bandages—one of paramedics administering emergency treatment or of unpleasant accidents. This is not a book that will tell you how to set a fracture, bandage a sprain or apply a tourniquet. It is about everyday plants—kitchen vegetables as well as more conventional medicinal herbs—that can be used to cope with the commonplace ailments that send us reaching into the household medicine chest. It is about herbal alternatives to over-the-counter cough drops, painkillers or other patent remedies and aims to highlight a few of the many ways in which we can use familiar plants. If you have nothing more on hand than a few apples, a cabbage, a jar of honey and an onion, then you will have a good selection of remedies to cope with many of the family's minor ailments. Add to that a jar of marigold or tea tree cream, homeopathic arnica tablets, a few slippery elm capsules, lavender oil—and a good selection of bandages—and you can handle almost any emergency.

Herbs for the First Aid Kit

In an age of painkilling sprays, instant burn relief creams and antiseptics guaranteed to "kill all known germs," traditional herbal first aid can sometimes seem medieval—to say the least. After all, in the modern housewife's larder of shrink-wrapped, precooked convenience meals, how many would easily find a fresh cabbage leaf to use for mastitis or swollen joints? How many could immediately lay their hands on raw onions to make a cough mixture or find fresh plantain growing in the garden to soothe insect bites?

Taken literally, the herbal first aid kit could look rather like a produce department's rejects. Fortunately, ready-made herbal alternatives to orthodox potions and liniments are readily accessible, while basic knowledge of the properties of a few common wayside plants usually means that for minor accidents, emergency remedies are close at hand.

The list of contents for the family's first aid kit starts with aloe vera, which will happily grow in a pot on the kitchen window sill and is ideal for all those minor burns cooking pots so frequently bestow on us, and ends with yarrow, a common weed and meadow herb which is ideal as an emergency treatment for nosebleeds.

Plant availability and space are the key limiting factors. If space is tight, buy the most versatile remedies that can be used for a wide range of ailments. For example, St. John's wort tincture can externally relieve cuts, scrapes, burns, inflammations and joint stiffness and internally can help with depression, insomnia, menstrual pains, neuralgia and immune disorders. If you are susceptible to frequent digestive disorders, headaches or muscle pains, your personal first aid kit can ease your distress quickly and effectively.

The 50 plants listed in this section are all suitable candidates for inclusion in the first aid kit. Some will be familiar as the popular herbs you can buy at the health food store or pharmacy, while others are more familiar as fruits or vegetables. Where accurate identification is important, detailed botanical descriptions are included for plants which may be gathered in the wild.

Unless quantities are specified, the standard proportions given in the next chapter should be used when making remedies.

Aloe   (Aloe vera)

Aloe is a tropical African plant which has been used medicinally since ancient times. In the West, the juice has traditionally been regarded as a soothing wound herb, but in Ayurvedic medicine it is treated as a restorative tonic. "Aloe vera" is also the commercial name given to the mucilaginous gel from one particular type of aloe which has become extremely popular in recent years both as a tonic remedy and as an ingredient in skin creams and cosmetic lotions.

Description: A perennial plant growing in clumps and producing numerous suckers or off-shoots. Leaves are thick and spiky with white splashes which appear red-tinged in young plants. Tubular flowers appear on long stems in summer.

Parts used: Leaves, sap.

Actions: Antifungal, anthelmintic, cholagogue, demulcent, purgative, styptic, sedative, tonic, wound healer.

Uses: As a bitter purgative, "bitter aloes" is widely included in over-the-counter remedies for constipation. Commercial aloe extracts are also sold as general tonics. For home first aid, use the gel (collected by opening a leaf and scraping out the sap) or the split fresh leaves applied directly, for scrapes, minor burns, eczema, sunburn, fungal infections such as ringworm and thrush and inflammations. To store a large quantity of sap, simmer it in a double boiler to produce a thick concentrate which can then be stored in jars.

Apple   (*Malus communis*)

Eating an apple a day to "keep the doctor away" is advice that many will remember from childhood. Today, researchers recommend apples for anti-cancer diets and to help lower blood cholesterol levels.

Part used: Fruit.

Actions: Antirheumatic, antiseptic, digestive and liver stimulant, diuretic, laxative, lowers cholesterol levels, tonic.

Uses: Unripe apples make an astringent remedy for diarrhea while ripe apples have a laxative effect. Traditionally apple juice and teas have been used as cooling remedies for fevers and inflammations including conjunctivitis (use well-diluted apple juice in an eyewash). Raw apples can be mashed and used as a soothing poultice for skin inflammations, while cooked apples are a traditional remedy for diarrhea and dysentery. A bowl of stewed apples will soothe gastritis.

Apricot   (*Prunus armeniaca*)

Apricots originate in China where the seeds are mainly used for treating asthma and bronchitis. The fruits are highly nutritious, very rich in vitamins A, B-complex and C and a good source of many essential minerals including iron, calcium and manganese.

Part used: Fruit.

Actions: Astringent, antianemic, immune stimulant, laxative, nutrient.

Uses: Apricots are rich in iron so can be helpful for iron-deficient anemia. When dried they are a laxative, while fresh apricots have an astringent effect. Eat fresh puréed apricots to combat diarrhea. Apricot oil is used as a skin softener while apricot jam is a traditional European nerve tonic used to combat insomnia and to strengthen a convalescing patient.

Arnica   (*Arnica montana*)

Also known as leopard's bane, this daisy-like alpine flower has a long history of use in central Europe as a remedy for bruises and sprains. A popular folk remedy for heart problems, it is still used in Germany for that purpose. However, since it is extremely toxic, internal use of arnica is restricted in many countries.

Description: A perennial growing to around 24 inches with golden-yellow daisy-like flowers up to two inches across. It grows from a basal rosette of oval-shaped, hairy leaves in summer.

Part used: Flowers.

Actions: Antibacterial, anti-inflammatory, astringent, bitter, heart stimulant, immune stimulant.

Uses: Arnica creams are readily available and make an essential home remedy for strains and bruises, chilblains (if the skin is unbroken) or painful varicose veins. It encourages the circulation to promote healing and tissue repair. Recent research also suggests that the herb may have immune-stimulant properties. As an internal remedy, arnica is used in homeopathic doses for shock, traumatic injury and to encourage healing after surgery. Take arnica 6x tablets (1 tablet every 30 minutes) after any major shock, accident, surgery or childbirth.

Cautions: Because of its toxicity, arnica should never be used on broken skin; in some cases it can cause contact dermatitis. It should be taken internally only in homeopathic doses; undiluted quantities can lead to palpitations, muscle paralysis and breathing problems and, in rare cases, may be fatal.

Bilberries and Cranberries (*Vaccinium* spp.)

Medicinal interest in bilberries (*V. myrtillus*) and their close relatives, cowberries (*V. vitis-idaea*) and cranberries (*V. macrocarpon*), has revived in recent years with work focussing on the use of cranberry juice as a cleansing diuretic in cystitis. These culinary berries are also closely related to bearberry (*Arctostaphylos uva-ursi*), an important urinary antiseptic. Cranberries, a North American fruit, were used by Native Americans in wound dressings.

Parts used: Leaves, berries.

Actions: Antibacterial, antiseptic, anti-emetic, astringent, hypoglycemic, tonic, high vitamin C content.

Uses: Elizabethan apothecaries made a syrup of bilberries with honey, called rob, which was used as a remedy for diarrhea. In large quantities, however, the berries are laxative and make a palatable treatment for constipation.

Externally, bilberries and cranberries can be used in creams and ointments for hemorrhoids, burns, minor wounds and skin complaints. Recent research has shown that the leaves will reduce blood sugar levels so they can be helpful in adult-onset diabetes that is under dietary control. The berries can be eaten stewed or fresh for digestive problems. Cranberry juice is ideal as a preventive for urinary infections for those prone to recurrent cystitis. Take ½ cup of the juice 3 times a day.

Cabbage (*Brassica oleracea*)

Jean Valnet, a notable French herbalist, has described cabbage as "the medicine of the poor," and it is probably one of the most widely used household remedies in folk tradition. The plant has been cultivated in the West since at least 400 B.C. and, in the second century A.D., the Greek herbalist Dioscorides considered it a digestive remedy, joint tonic and cooling preparation for skin problems and fevers. In Germany, sauerkraut, a fermented cabbage mixture, is regarded as a preventive for cancer, rheumatism, gout and premature aging.

Part used: Whole plant.

Actions: Anti-inflammatory, antibacterial, antirheumatic, liver decongestant, tissue proliferant and healing.

Uses: The leaves have been used as anti-inflammatory poultices to relieve inflammatory complaints ranging from arthritis to mastitis, while cabbage lotions were once a regular household standby for skin problems. Cabbage juices and infusions are used to treat a range of digestive problems including stomach ulcers.

The fresh leaves can be applied directly to inflammations (simply soften them with a vegetable mallet and secure with a loose bandage or Band-Aid). A crushed cabbage leaf inserted between breast and bra is a simple but very effective remedy for mastitis when breast feeding. A useful lotion for acne can be made by combining cabbage leaves and distilled witch hazel in a food processor.

Cayenne (*Capsicum frutescens*)

Various chili species are used medicinally including *C. frutescens* and the hot pepper used in cooking, *C. annuum*. Cayenne became extremely popular in the 19th century with the Physiomedicalists, a group of traditional healers who lived in New England. The herb increases perspiration and was used in the ''sweating'' treatments favored by the Physiomedicalists which were based on the Native American tradition of sweat lodges.

Part used: Fruit.

Actions: Antiseptic, antibacterial, carminative, circulatory stimulant, diaphoretic, gastric stimulant; topically: counterirritant, rubefacient.

Uses: Many Western herbalists still add cayenne to mixtures for treating ''cold'' complaints such as arthritis, digestive weakness and general debility, and the herb is regarded as a useful stimulant for both the digestion and circulation. Externally, cayenne ointments can be used to encourage blood flow and may be helpful for treating chilblains, lumbago, muscle pain, the pain of shingles, and nerve pains like neuralgia. It can be made into a hot infused oil (use about 2 tablespoons of dried chili to 1 quart of sunflower oil) which can be used directly as a lotion or thickened with beeswax to make an ointment.

Chamomile (*Matricaria recutita/Chamaemelum nobile*)

Both German chamomile (*M. recutita*) and its relative, Roman chamomile (*C. nobile*), are among the most widely used of medicinal herbs. Their actions are very similar, although Roman chamomile has a slightly more bitter taste and German chamomile is somewhat more effective as an anti-inflammatory and analgesic. While herbalists may have their individual favorites, the plants are extremely close in action and can be regarded as interchangeable in lay use.

Description: Sweetly scented annual, biennial or perennial plant with many branched stems and finely divided leaves. Flowers are daisy-like.

Parts used: Flowers, essential oil.

Actions: Anti-emetic, anti-inflammatory, antispasmodic, bitter, carminative, sedative.

Uses: Both types of chamomile can be taken internally in teas for nervous stomach upsets, nausea or insomnia, and they can be made into creams for external use on eczema, wounds, diaper rash, sore nipples and piles. The infusion can also be used as a steam inhalation for catarrh, sinus problems and to help control mild asthma attacks.

Chamomile is also used in homeopathy. Chamomilla 3x pellets and drops make a valuable standby for babies to treat both colic and teething. It is one of the safest herbs for children and babies; weak infusions (¼ to ½ normal strength depending on the child's age) can be given as a night-time drink to encourage restful sleep. The infusion can also be added to bath water to soothe overexcited infants.

Chamomile yields a deep blue essential oil on steam distillation which is both very relaxing and useful in skin care: add 2 to 3 drops to bathwater to soothe emotional problems. It is also useful in bathwater for muscle aches and pain. For joint inflammations and swellings (including tennis elbow) soak a cloth in a diluted mixture (5 drops in a cup of water) and use as a cold compress. For digestive disorders make a massage oil using 5 drops in 1 tablespoon of almond oil and use to rub the abdomen.

Chickweed (*Stellaria media*)

Chickweed, as the name suggests, is a favorite food for domestic fowl. It is an extremely common garden weed which can be cooked like spinach and tossed in butter or used as a salad herb.

Description: A spreading, low-growing annual with brittle stems and well-spaced oval leaves. Small, white, star-like flowers appear throughout the year.

Parts used: Aerial parts.

Actions: Antirheumatic, astringent, demulcent, wound herb, contains vitamin C.

Uses: Chickweed is soothing and astringent; its main medicinal use is in creams and ointments for irritant skin rashes and eczema or for burns, boils and drawing splinters. The whole flowering chickweed plant can also easily be made into an infused oil (using the hot method, p. 56) and added to bathwater to soothe skin problems. Use 2 teaspoons of the infused oil in a warm bath. Although not so popular as an internal remedy, it is cleansing and antirheumatic and can be made into a tea to help ease rheumatic aches and pains.

Cinnamon   (*Cinnamomum zeylanicum*)

Cinnamon is widely used as a flavoring in cooking although it also has a long tradition as a medicinal plant. The Chinese regard cinnamon twigs as warming for the peripheries and use them to encourage circulation to cold hands and feet, while the inner bark is seen as more centrally warming and is used to treat cold problems associated with low energy such as debility, rheumatic problems and kidney weakness.

Parts used: Inner bark, twigs.

Actions: Antispasmodic, antiseptic, carminative, warming digestive remedy, diaphoretic, tonic; topical essential oil: antibacterial and antifungal.

Uses: As a warming herb, cinnamon can be helpful for all sorts of "cold" conditions including chills and rheumatic pains. Add a pinch of powdered cinnamon to teas to make a soothing drink to combat colds, chills, aches or stomach upsets or combine it with ginger in a warming decoction. (Mix 1 slice of fresh ginger root and a 2-inch length of cinnamon bark to 1½ cups of water.) Cinnamon has been used for centuries to treat nausea and vomiting and is also helpful for many digestive problems including diarrhea and gastroenteritis. The herb also shows some antifungal activity and is sometimes added to remedies for candidiasis.

Caution: Cinnamon should be avoided in pregnancy.

Cloves (*Syzygium aromaticum*)

Cloves have been used for flavoring for around 2,000 years and were known in Roman times as an exotic spice. The Chinese have used them medicinally since around 600 A.D., regarding them as a kidney tonic to increase *yang* energy and treat impotence. The herb is familiar as a culinary spice, a traditional favorite with baked apples.

Parts used: Flower buds, essential oil.

Actions: Mild anaesthetic, anodyne, anti-emetic, antiseptic, antispasmodic, carminative, warming stimulant.

Uses: Clove oil is available from many pharmacies and is useful as an emergency first aid remedy for toothache (put a few drops on a cotton swab and place on the gum nearest to the aching tooth). Cloves are useful for disguising the taste of more unpleasant herbs, so a couple of the dried flower buds added to an herbal mixture for stomach upsets or chills can often make the brew more palatable. In many parts of the East, clove oil is also used for abdominal massage during labor to encourage contractions and ease pain. Drinking teas flavored with plenty of cloves during the second stage of labor can help to ease childbirth pains.

Caution: Cloves should be reserved for labor and childbirth and not taken earlier in pregnancy.

Coffee (*Coffea arabica*)

Originally grown in Ethiopia, coffee production spread throughout the Arab world, reached Western Europe in the 17th century and was then introduced into South America by settlers. It is now one of the world's most important cash crops. Millions drink cups of it every day, and an entire industry has emerged to produce the necessary equipment for processing—percolators, espresso machines, filters and the like.

Part used: Beans.

Actions: Anti-emetic, antinarcotic, diuretic, stimulant.

Uses: Coffee's best known medicinal action is as a stimulant: it is rich in caffeine (3 parts per 1,000) which stimulates the central nervous system and increases heart rate. This in turn speeds blood flow through the kidneys, which explains coffee's mild diuretic action.

Palpitations are a common side effect of too much coffee drinking. In home first aid, coffee can be used to counter nausea and vomiting (much appreciated by hangover sufferers) and is worth remembering as a digestive stimulant which can increase gastrointestinal activity. In folk medicine the powdered beans have also been used as an emergency application to burns and scalds to control inflammation. In homeopathic doses, coffee has the opposite effect and is used for anxiety, stress, nervous headaches and hyperactivity.

Comfrey   (*Symphytum officinale*)

Although comfrey has been used for centuries as a wound healer and restorer of broken bones, it has had a more checkered history in recent years, veering from panacea to health hazard. Its healing action is due to a chemical called allantoin, which encourages growth of various tissue cells and so accelerates healing. Generations used comfrey poultices on pulled ligaments and minor fractures, while herbalists recommended it internally for stomach ulceration.

Description: Tall (up to 4 feet) perennial with stout stems and thick, hairy, tapering leaves. Flowers are white to purple and funnel-shaped, appearing in summer.

Parts used: Roots, leaves.

Actions: Astringent, cell proliferator, demulcent, expectorant, wound herb.

Uses: Comfrey is ideal used externally for any sort of tissue damage. The hot infused oil is easy to make and forms a useful base for massage rubs for bruises, strains, sprains and similar traumatic injuries; add 5 drops of rosemary or lavender essential oil to 1 teaspoon of comfrey infused oil. Many herbalists suggest that regular gentle massage using comfrey oil (for six to eight weeks) can help repair the damage of old injuries which may contribute to osteoarthritis. The herb should not be used on fresh wounds before they are thoroughly cleaned since the rapid healing caused by the allantoin may trap dirt, leading to abscesses.

Cautions: During the 1960s and 1970s the plant became overhyped as a cure-all for arthritis, and this inevitably focussed research interest on its constituents. Researchers fed large amounts of the plant to rats which subsequently died of liver disorders, and comfrey's pyrrolizidine alkaloids were blamed. Comfrey supporters argue that the rats had so much comfrey to eat they actually suffered from the effects of malnutrition. Some also maintain that only small amounts of the alkaloids are extracted in conventional herbal preparations (infusions and ointments) so that these are quite safe in normal low doses, although this has not been confirmed in tests.[1] Health authorities have tended to disagree. Comfrey is now banned in many parts of the world; where it is not banned, some advise against using it on open wounds. Traditionally, comfrey was never used as a long-term medication; it was regarded as an external treatment for short-term use only. If we follow this convention, many herbalists consider it no more toxic than any other form of medication.

Cucumber   (*Cucumis sativus*)

Cucumbers are cleansing, diuretic and refreshing, help to dissolve uric acid and thus are useful for gout and arthritis. Cucumbers are around 95 percent water but do contain vitamins A, B-complex and C as well as manganese, sulphur and other minerals.

Parts used: Fruit.

Actions: Cleansing, cooling, diuretic, clears uric acid.

Uses: Cool slices of cucumber are useful as eye pads to soothe tired and inflamed eyes, while internally they can cool the stomach and thus are a useful food to eat for gastric irritations and colic. Lightly cooked cucumber is best for digestive problems.

Cucumbers are also a favorite with beauticians as the basis for moisturizers and other skin products. A home-made alternative is simply to purée a peeled cucumber in the food processor and store the resulting liquid in the refrigerator for use as a lotion. The same mixture is ideal to soothe sunburn and minor skin irritations or you can use thin slices as a poultice. Cucumber lotions or poultices can also be helpful for enlarged pores, oily skin, wrinkles and skin blemishes and are also soothing for insect stings, cold sores and prickly heat.

Echinacea   (*Echinacea angustifolia, E. pallida, E. purpurea*)

Echinacea, or purple coneflower, was one of the most important herbs used by Native American healers. The herb was treated as a universal antidote to snake bite, the juice was used to bathe burns, and pieces of root were chewed for toothache. By the 1850s echinacea was already widely used by European settlers, largely as an aromatic and carminative for digestive problems.

Interest in the plant spread and, by the 1930s, research in Germany had highlighted its potent antibiotic actions. Although the roots of various related species are generally used medicinally, work in Germany[2] suggests that the aerial parts of *E. purpurea* are more efficacious than its root, which makes the plant ideal for garden cultivation and regular cropping.

Description: A tall (up to 4 feet) perennial with slim, lanceolate leaves and large, daisy-like purple flowers with well-separated, dropping petals. Centers are red-brown and conical, hence the common name "purple coneflower."

Parts used: Root, aerial parts.

Actions: Antibiotic, anti-allergenic, anti-inflammatory, immune stimulant, lymphatic tonic, vulnerary.

Uses: Echinacea is the ideal remedy for any sort of infection such as colds, influenza, boils, wounds, septicemia, kidney or urinary tract infections. For general use, it is best to take echinacea in high doses at the first sign of a cold using 2 teaspoons of a 1:5 tincture, or 3 200-mg capsules, 3 times daily for up to 4 days. Studies confirm that higher doses are most effective for upper-respiratory tract infections with a minimum dose of 2 teaspoons of tincture a day needed for significant improvements in upper-respiratory tract problems.[3] The herb is also helpful for general immune deficiency where there are recurrent infections.

Echinacea creams can be helpful for skin infections, cuts and scrapes. In severe cases it is best to support the external remedy with additional echinacea taken internally. Although most herbalists suggest that echinacea is best taken in short sharp bursts of up to four weeks, others regard it as a prophylactic and will happily recommend low dosages to school-age children on a long-term basis to successfully prevent the usual round of childhood ills (1 200-mg capsule daily).

Elder   (*Sambucus nigra*)

In the Middle Ages, many people believed that the elder tree was inhabited by a spirit known as the "elder mother" whose permission was needed if ever the tree was to be pruned; thus felling elders was considered a guarantee of bad luck, although branches from the tree placed over doors and windows were believed to keep witches away and ward off the Evil Eye. Such respect was understandable since the elder is almost a complete medicine chest. The leaves are the basis of a green ointment for sprains and strains, the inner bark is a strong purgative, the berries (a good source of vitamin C) act as a prophylactic against colds and infections, while the flowers are strongly anti-catarrhal.

Description: A large shrubby tree with pinnate leaves and tiny, scented cream flowers borne in flat bunches in early summer. The dark purple berries ripen in late autumn.

Parts used: Flowers collected in spring and berries in autumn; the bark, leaves and root have all been used in the past. Collect the leaves in summer after flowering.

Actions: Anti-inflammatory, anticatarrhal, diaphoretic, diuretic, emollient (flowers), laxative (berries and bark).

Uses: Today we mainly use elder flowers as a soothing anticatarrhal and diaphoretic remedy, although they are also topically anti-inflammatory and emollient and make a very effective hand cream. Elder flower water (made by distilling the flowers) was a favorite in the 18th century for whitening the skin and removing freckles. Elder flowers also appear to strengthen the mucous membranes so can increase resistance to irritant allergens. Drinking elder flower tea in early spring can help reduce hay fever symptoms later in the year. A hot infused oil of elder leaves also makes a useful green ointment for bruises and minor injuries.

Eucalyptus   (*Eucalyptus globulus*)

The majority of eucalyptus species originated in Australia where the plant was widely used in Aboriginal medicine to treat fevers, dysentery and sores. In the 19th century, the plant was brought to Europe, and cultivation of the tree spread in Southern Europe and North America.

Parts used: Leaves, essential oil.

Actions: Antiseptic, antispasmodic, anthelmintic, expectorant, febrifuge, lowers blood sugar levels, stimulant.

Uses: Eucalyptus oil (extracted by steam distillation) is ideal for home use and is mainly used externally in rubs for muscle aches and steam inhalations for catarrh and colds. For rubs use up to 5 drops of essential oil in 1 teaspoon of a vegetable or almond oil base; add 5 drops to a basin of boiling water for use in steam inhalations. The lemon-scented eucalyptus (*E. citriodora*) is antifungal and can be effective externally for athlete's foot and other fungal infections.

Caution: Excess use may cause headache and delirium. Do not take eucalyptus oil internally.

Eyebright   (*Euphrasia officinalis*)

Eyebright is one of our most effective anti-catarrhals and, as the name suggests, a favorite eye remedy. It was first mentioned in the 14th century as a cure for "all evils of the eye."

Description: An annual, low-growing plant with upright, rounded, toothed leaves and small white three-lobed flowers often streaked with purple and with a yellow throat.

Parts used: Aerial parts.

Actions: Anticatarrhal, anti-inflammatory, astringent, tonic.

Uses: Eyebright is useful for both hay fever and common colds. It can be taken in teas (2 teaspoons to 1 cup of water) or powdered in capsules (3 200-mg capsules up to 3 times a day). It is also a good soothing remedy for many eye infections and irritations. It is best to use decoctions rather than infusions for eyewashes to ensure that the mixture is quite sterile. Use 3 heaped teaspoons of the herb to 2 cups of boiling water and simmer gently until the mixture has been reduced by about ⅓. Strain the mix well and allow to cool thoroughly before using. Alternatively soak a small clean linen cloth in the infusion and use as a compress applied to the affected eye while still warm. Because of its astringent qualities, eyebright infusion can also be used as a gargle for sore throats and hoarseness.

Evening Primrose (*Oenotheris biennis*)

A native of North America, evening primrose is now widely naturalized across Europe. The leaves were traditionally used for asthma and digestive disorders; however, during the 1970s researchers found that the seeds are rich in an essential fatty acid called gamma-linolenic acid (GLA) that is vital for good health.

Description: A tall (up to 5 feet) biennial with a basal rosette of pointed leaves and scattered leaves on the stems. In summer large, pale yellow flowers, which have a heavy scent in the evenings, appear along the stem, giving a prolonged flowering period.

Part used: Seed oil.

Action: Alterative, hormone regulator, source of essential fatty acids.

Uses: GLA is reputed to ease menstrual and menopausal problems, strengthen the circulatory system, combat certain sorts of eczema and boost the immune system. Research suggests that it can ease irritable bowel syndrome when symptoms are associated with the menstrual cycle. In clinical trials dosages of 3 to 5 g a day have been commonplace although commercial capsules generally contain 250 to 1000 mg and most suppliers recommend 500 to 1000 mg a day. The oil can also be used on the skin for eczema and similar problems. Because evening primrose oil helps to normalize liver function it can be useful to counter the symptoms of a hangover on "the morning after." Take up to 2 g of the oil in capsules.

Fennel   (*Foeniculum officinalis*)

Fennel has been cultivated since Roman times for its thick bulbous stems which are eaten as a vegetable, as well as its feathery leaves, which are used for flavoring, and its seeds, which have medicinal benefits.

Part used: Seeds; the stem base is eaten as a vegetable.

Actions: Anti-inflammatory, carminative, circulatory stimulant, diuretic, mild expectorant, galactogogue.

Uses: Fennel seed tea is ideal for indigestion, gas or colic and can be added to laxative mixtures to ease the griping pains that strong purgatives can cause. Fennel tea bags are readily available and make a good after-dinner drink to ease the digestion. Fennel tea also makes a good mouthwash for gum disease and sore throats and is sometimes included in herbal toothpastes. Fennel is used in commercial remedies to ease baby's colic, although an alternative for breastfeeding mothers would be simply to drink fennel infusion a couple of hours before feeding so that the baby receives its medicinal herbs with the daily milk. The essential oil is sold commercially and can be added to external rubs for bronchial congestion; use 5 drops of oil in a teaspoon of almond oil.

Feverfew   (*Tanacetum parthenium*)

Feverfew has hit the media headlines in recent years as a major "cure" and prophylactic for migraine and arthritis. Since the 1970s, the plant has been extensively researched and is known to contain parthenolides and similar compounds which are believed to account for its action. Although there was some traditional use of feverfew for headaches, this was largely in external applications.

Description: A perennial with daisy-like flowers borne in clusters on stems with yellow-green lobed leaves. Plants are bushy and grow to around 24 inches in height.

Part used: Leaves.

Actions: Anti-inflammatory, analgesic, antispasmodic, anthelmintic, cooling, digestive stimulant, emmenagogue, peripheral vasodilator, relaxant.

Uses: Chewing a fresh feverfew leaf each day is believed by many to prevent migraines. The tea can be useful for acute arthritic attacks and, as an antispasmodic, it can be helpful for menstrual pain.

Caution: Feverfew shows antiplatelet activity (reduces the blood's clotting ability) so should not be used by those taking warfarin, heparin and similar blood-thinning drugs. Migraine sufferers should stop taking regular doses of feverfew if side effects (skin rashes or mouth ulceration) occur.

Garlic   (*Allium sativa*)

Garlic is one of mankind's oldest medicinal herbs; recipes using the plant have been found in the cuneiform script of ancient Babylon dating back at least 5,000 years. Its characteristic smell is due to a group of sulphur-containing compounds, notably allicin, which account for its medicinal activity. Deodorizing garlic by removing the allicin thus makes the remedy markedly less effective.

Part used: Clove.

Actions: Antibiotic, antihistamine, antiparasitic, antithrombotic, diaphoretic, expectorant, hypotensive, reduces cholesterol levels, reduces blood sugar levels.

Uses: Garlic has been used since ancient times as a remedy for colds, chest infections and digestive upsets, including amoebic dysentery; today we know it is strongly antibacterial and antifungal, thus active against a wide spectrum of infections. It also reduces cholesterol levels in the blood, helping to prevent the development of arteriosclerosis.

In the East, garlic has long been regarded as an important tonic for the elderly, helping to improve weak digestive function, and researchers have now shown that low doses of garlic (typically a daily clove used in cooking) do indeed have a tonifying effect on the intestine, improving peristalsis and performance. For colds and catarrhal problems take up to 2 g of garlic in capsule form daily. If using fresh garlic, mash 1 clove and mix with ½ cup of hot milk to make a pungent, but palatable drink. Repeat up to 3 times a day. Eating parsley can help to reduce garlic odor.

Caution: High doses of garlic are best avoided in pregnancy and lactation as they may lead to heartburn or flavor breast milk.

Ginger   (*Zingiber officinalis*)

Ginger originated in tropical Asia and spread to Europe in ancient times; it is mentioned by the Romans, listed in some of the earliest Chinese herbals, regarded in Ayurvedic medicine as a universal medicine, and introduced by the Spaniards to America where it is now cultivated extensively in the West Indies. It has a pungent, aromatic flavor and is widely used as a commercial flavoring. As a hot, dry herb it was traditionally used to warm the stomach and dispel chills.

Part used: Root.

Actions: Anti-emetic, antiseptic, antispasmodic, carminative, circulatory stimulant, diaphoretic, expectorant, peripheral vasodilator; topically: rubefacient.

Uses: Ginger is ideal in warming decoctions for colds and chills. Simply use the fresh ginger from the grocery store and simmer 1 to 2 slices in 1½ cups of water as a decoction or add a pinch of powdered ginger to other herb teas. As a remedy for nausea, ginger is ideal for travel sickness and has been very successfully tested in clinical trials for severe morning sickness in pregnancy (typical dose is up to 1 g of powdered herb, roughly equal to a level teaspoon, 3 times a day).[4] Ginger in capsules is ideal, but ginger snaps or ginger ale can also prove effective, especially with children.

Ginger oil is used in external remedies to encourage blood flow to ease muscular stiffness, aches and pains; a suitable home-made substitute is to add 1 tablespoon of chopped fresh ginger to 2 cups of sunflower oil and heat in a double saucepan over water for 3 hours. Strain and store the oil, when cool, in a dark place; use as a massage rub. In Chinese medicine fresh and dried root are regarded rather differently, with the dried root believed to be more helpful for abdominal pain and diarrhea and the fresh root more suitable for feverish chills, coughs and vomiting.

Honey

Although not an herb, honey is such a useful and readily available first aid remedy that it certainly deserves its place in this list. Honey is rich in sugars, vitamins B and C, calcium, iron, magnesium, silica and other mineral salts and is a nutritious and soothing food for debility and convalescence.

Actions: Antiseptic, expectorant, soothing demulcent.

Uses: Honey has a long-standing reputation as a cough and catarrh remedy, and mixtures of honey and lemon are still widely available over the counter. It is ideal to use in cough syrups (see p. 55), and adding a teaspoon of honey to a cup of hot lemon juice is an ideal remedy for sore throats, coughs and colds. It can also be helpful for hay fever and allergic rhinitis; try an eyebright infusion (2 teaspoons of herb to 1 cup of water) mixed with 2 teaspoons of honey.

Honey makes a useful base for taking herb powders; simply mix a level teaspoon of the herb powder with 3 teaspoons of honey and take in teaspoon doses during the day. This can often prove an efficient way of persuading small children (and their fathers) to swallow their medicine. Honey is a potent antiseptic and can be applied externally to wounds, sores and abscesses. It is useful for bringing boils to a head and can be soothing for minor burns and inflammations. Apply a little directly to the affected area and cover with gauze.

Cautions: Unpasteurized honey should not be given internally to children under the age of 18 months.

Juniper   (*Juniperis communis*)

Traditionally juniper berries have been associated with sacred cleansing rituals, and sprigs of the plant are still regularly burned each day in Tibetan temples as part of the morning purification rite. The Egyptians used the berries in mummification, and several medicinal recipes survive in Egyptian papyri dating back to 1550 BC.

Parts used: Berries, essential oil.

Actions: Anti-inflammatory, antirheumatic, antiseptic, carminative, digestive tonic, diuretic, urinary antiseptic, uterine stimulant.

Uses: Juniper berries are widely used for urinary tract problems, such as cystitis, and as a cleansing remedy for rheumatism. For home use the essential oil, collected by steam-distilling the berries, is more practical and can be used as a stimulating massage for muscular aches and pains. Use 10 drops of juniper oil to 1 tablespoon of almond oil and massage affected areas every 2 to 3 hours. An essential oil is also made from dry-distilling the heartwood of various juniper species. Known as ''cade oil'' this substance is highly aromatic and antiseptic and is a useful remedy for various skin problems. Add 20 drops to 1 quart of hot water and use as a hair rinse for dandruff, scaling eczema or psoriasis affecting the scalp.

Caution: Prolonged use of juniper can irritate the kidneys, and any preparation containing the herb should not be taken internally for longer than six weeks without professional advice. It should not be taken internally at all by those suffering from kidney disease, and high doses must be avoided in pregnancy.

Lavender   (*Lavandula angustifolia*)

Lavender has been used to scent baths and toiletries since Roman times. In Arabic medicine, the herb is still used today as an expectorant and remedy for chest problems.

Description: A flowering shrub with downy, pointed grey-green leaves and tall stems (up to 15 inches long) bearing tiny lilac to purple flowers.

Parts used: Flowers, essential oil.

Actions: Analgesic, antibacterial, antidepressant, antispasmodic, carminative, cholagogue, circulatory stimulant, relaxant, tonic for the nervous system.

Uses: Lavender is useful for digestive upsets, nervous tension, insomnia, migraines and headaches. The flowers can be made into a pleasant-tasting tea taken at night for sleeplessness or during the day for headaches and nervous tension. The same tea will also help to cool feverish conditions, encouraging sweating and thus lowering the body temperature. Use 2 teaspoons of lavender flowers to a cup of boiling water and sweeten with a little honey if required. An essential oil can be steam-distilled from the flowers and is a vital member of the first aid kit. Use it diluted (add 10 drops of lavender oil to 1 teaspoon of sunflower or almond oil) as a massage for muscular aches and pains or massage gently into the temples and nape of the neck to relieve tension headaches and migraines.

The same amount of lavender in an infused St. John's

wort oil base makes a soothing lotion for sunburn and minor scalds and it can also help deter insects if applied to exposed skin. Added to bath water, 5 drops of lavender oil make a relaxing and soothing soak for nervous tension and insomnia, and you can also add 5 drops to a basin of boiling water for use as a steam inhalation to clear catarrh. The oil can be diluted in warm water (20 drops to half a quart) and used as an antiseptic wash for scrapes and cuts.

Lemon   (*Citrus limonum*)

Lemons were considered by the Romans as an antidote for poisons, and in modern Italy eating fresh lemons is still believed, by many, to combat major epidemic infections. They are certainly very rich in minerals and vitamins, including B_1, B_2, B_3, carotene (pro-vitamin A), and C.

Parts used: Fruit, essential oil.

Actions: Antibacterial, anti-inflammatory, antihistamine, antirheumatic, antiscorbutic, antiseptic, antiviral, carminative, cleansing, cooling, diuretic, tonifying for heart and blood vessels.

Uses: Lemons can improve the peripheral circulation and, as a venous tonic, may be helpful for hemorrhoids and varicose veins. In folk medicine, lemons have always been a popular remedy for feverish chills and coughs, and numerous over-the-counter products based on honey and lemon mixtures are widely available. A home-made alternative is to combine the juice of 2 lemons with 1 teaspoon of honey and a cup of hot water, stir well and drink 3 times a day.

An essential oil can be distilled from the fruit. To avoid concentrating pesticide residues, it is advisable to use organically-grown lemons for this purpose. Lemon oil diluted in water (or warm lemon juice) makes a good gargle for sore throats. Lemon diluted in sunflower or almond oil can be used to relieve insect stings and the pain of neuralgia. Simply rub a little directly on the affected area. Fresh lemon juice or slices of lemon make an acceptable alternative in both cases.

Externally, lemon juice can also be used to ease sunburn and irritating skin rashes. As a styptic (stops bleeding) it can be used on cotton swabs to speed clotting in nosebleeds and it will make an emergency antiseptic wash for cuts and scrapes. Press a swab soaked in juice directly onto cuts.

Lemon is also popular in traditional beauty treatments to whiten the skin and the teeth and to encourage freckles to fade. Mixed with equal amounts of glycerine and eau de cologne, lemon juice makes a soothing and softening hand lotion. Rotten lemons can be used to repel ants.

Lemon Balm   (*Melissa officinalis*)

Lemon balm has a long association with bees and the healing power of their products. It was regarded by the Greeks as a cure-all.

Description: A lemon-scented perennial plant with oval, toothed leaves on square stems growing to around 3 feet. Flowers are insignificant and appear in axils in clusters in summer.

Parts used: Aerial parts, essential oil.

Actions: Antibacterial, antidepressant, antiviral, diaphoretic, digestive stimulant, peripheral vasodilator, relaxing restorative for nervous system, sedative.

Uses: A carminative and sedative, lemon balm is

useful to reduce body temperature in fevers and to treat nervous tummy upsets in children. It is, however, potent enough to help with depression, anxiety and tension headaches.

The herb grows easily in most climates, and an infusion made from a handful of fresh leaves to a cup of boiling water makes a refreshing and restorative drink at the end of the day. For winter use it needs to be dried quickly to avoid losing too much of the characteristic lemon flavor. If using dried lemon balm add 2 teaspoons of the herb to each cup of boiling water.

Externally, lemon balm cream or infused oil can be used on insect bites, sores and slow-healing wounds. The essential oil is available commercially and used in aromatherapy as a massage for nervous problems. For a relaxing massage oil, add 2 to 3 drops of the oil to a teaspoon of almond or sunflower oil. It also makes a good insect repellent: put 20 drops of oil into 1 quart of water and use in a hand spray.

Licorice   (*Glycyrrhiza glabra*)

Licorice is one of our most widely researched and respected medicinal herbs; it has been used since at least 500 B.C. and drugs based on licorice extracts are still listed in official pharmacopoeias as remedies for gastric ulcers and inflammation. In traditional Chinese herbalism it is called the "great detoxifier" or "great harmonizer" and is believed to drive toxins and poisons from the system and eliminate the harmful side effects of other herbs. Licorice has a hormonal effect, stimulating the adrenal cortex and encouraging production of such hormones as hydrocortisone.

Part used: Root.

Actions: Antiarthritic, anti-inflammatory, antispasmodic, cooling, lowers cholesterol levels, expectorant, mild laxative, soothing for gastric mucosa, tonic stimulant for adrenal cortex, possibly antiallergenic.

Uses: Licorice is very soothing and demulcent, making it ideal for gastric ulceration, and it is also a digestive stimulant and laxative helpful for constipation. Mix licorice root decoction (made by combining a tablespoon of dried root with 3 cups of water and simmering for 20 minutes) with a tablespoon of honey to make an effective cough syrup or take a tablespoon dose of the decoction as a tonic once a day. The same decoction can be combined with meadowsweet infusion (use equal amounts of each) as a remedy for gastritis, acidity and heartburn.

Caution: Excessive licorice can cause fluid retention and increase blood pressure and it should therefore be avoided by anyone suffering from hypertension. It should not be taken by those on digoxin-based drugs.

Marigold   (*Calendula officinalis*)

Pot marigolds have been among the herbalist's favorites for centuries.

Description: An annual flower with bright yellow or orange flowers in single or double rays. Stems are branched with pointed leaves and grow to around 20 inches.

Part used: Flowers.

Actions: Astringent, antiseptic, antifungal, anti-inflammatory, antispasmodic, bitter, cholagogue, diaphoretic, immune stimulant, menstrual regulator, wound herb.

Uses: Over-the-counter marigold creams are often

sold under the Latin name of *Calendula* and are an ideal antiseptic remedy for cuts, scrapes, fungal infections (including athlete's foot and vaginal yeast infection), minor burns and skin disorders such as dry eczema. Internally the herb can be used in infusions (3 teaspoons of petals to a cup of boiling water) as a bitter to stimulate bile production and improve the digestion. The same tea, taken 3 times daily, is ideal for a number of gynecological problems, including irregular or painful menstruation, and it can also be used for gastric and gallbladder inflammations and as a cleansing remedy for inflamed lymph glands.

The infusion can also be used as an antiseptic wash to bathe cuts and scrapes. For conjunctivitis, styes and other eye inflammations, use a well-strained and cooled decoction (made from 1 tablespoon of petals with 2 cups of water and simmered for 20 minutes) for a sterile eyewash.

A cold infused oil (p. 57) can easily be made at home using the fresh or dried flowers, and this makes a good alternative to commercial ointments or can be used as a base for essential oils. A strongly antifungal lotion for athlete's foot can be made by adding 5 drops of tea tree oil to a tablespoon of infused marigold oil. The infused oil can also be used directly on dry skin, or a tablespoon can be added to the bath water to ease irritant eczema. It also makes an antiseptic lotion for minor cuts and scrapes. The cream is helpful for soothing sore nipples in breast-feeding, an old-fashioned remedy which many maternity wards have now revived.

Meadowsweet   (*Filipendula ulmaria*)

Meadowsweet's best known claim to fame is as the

herb which gave us the name "aspirin." In the 1830s chemists first identified salicylic acid, extracted from willow bark, as an anti-inflammatory and analgesic. Over the following years they worked to produce a synthetic drug. By the 1890s, the German drug company Bayer had finally patented the result and, since salicylates extracted from meadowsweet had been involved in the development work, they named the drug "aspirin" after the old botanical name for meadowsweet, *Spiraea ulmaria*.

Description: A hardy perennial growing to around four feet in height and generally found in damp ditches and hedgerows. The plant has irregular pinnate leaves and large, fluffy, creamy flower heads that appear from midsummer to early autumn which smell slightly of aspirin.

Parts used: Whole plant collected when flowering.

Actions: Mild analgesic, antacid, anti-inflammatory, antirheumatic, antiseptic, astringent, diaphoretic, diuretic, soothing for the gastric membranes.

Uses: Meadowsweet was traditionally used in much the same way as we now use aspirin—as a remedy for easing pains and feverish colds and as an anti-inflammatory for arthritic conditions. Unlike aspirin, which can irritate the gastric lining and in prolonged use lead to ulceration, meadowsweet is extremely soothing and calming for the digestive tract. It is ideal for gastritis, indigestion and heartburn and is sometimes even described as having antiulcer activity. Make an infusion using 2 teaspoons of the dried herb to a cup of boiling water for each dose and take up to 3 times daily. Meadowsweet infusion is ideal for many minor stomach upsets and, taken after meals, is helpful to counter indigestion; for digestive problems it combines well with lemon balm (see p. 77).

Strong extracts of meadowsweet are used by professional herbalists in treating arthritis and rheumatism, although in mild cases a home-made infusion can be useful. Increase the proportions to up to 2 heaped tablespoons of dried herb to 3 cups of boiling water to make 3 doses.

Caution: Meadowsweet is best avoided by those sensitive to salicylates and aspirin.

Mustard   (*Brassica nigra/Sinapis alba*)

White mustard seeds (*Sinapis alba*) are larger in size than black mustard seeds (*Brassica nigra*) and tend to have a milder flavor. Both varieties are, however, used in very similar ways.

Parts used: Seeds.

Actions: Counterirritant, diaphoretic, diuretic, emetic, topically rubefacient.

Uses: Mustard foot baths, an effective means of stimulating the circulation and digestive systems, are also a traditional remedy for colds and chills. By encouraging blood flow to the feet, they can be helpful in reducing over-all body temperature by dissipating heat, and will also draw blood to the peripheries to combat chilblains. Use a tablespoon of mustard powder or seeds, preferably in a muslin bag, to 1 quart of hot water and soak the feet for 10 to 15 minutes.

Both black and white mustard seeds can be made into hot infused oils (often combined with cayenne) to make a warming rub for muscular stiffness, aches and pains. Use 1 tablespoon of mustard seeds to 3 cups of sunflower oil and heat in a double boiler for 2 hours.

Caution: Mustards can irritate the skin, and prolonged use of poultices can lead to blistering.

Oats

(*Avena sativa*)

Oats are one of the world's most important cereal crops; they have been used as a staple food in northern Europe for centuries. As a food, oats are sweet, nutritious and warming—ideal to combat cold, damp climates—and form the basis of porridge, once the staple food of generations of Scottish highlanders. Oats are rich in iron, zinc and manganese, thus a good source of many vital minerals.

Parts used: Seeds and grain extracts, whole plant.

Actions: Oatstraw: antidepressant, restorative nerve tonic, diaphoretic; seeds: antidepressant, restorative nerve tonic, nutritive; bran: antithrombotic, lowers cholesterol levels; fresh plant: antirheumatic in homeopathic tincture.

Uses: Since oats are an antidepressant, a restorative nerve tonic and emotionally uplifting, a bowl of hot cereal made from good quality oatmeal is the ideal way to start the day. Extracts of the whole plant (the oatstraw) are generally used by herbalists, with the tincture prescribed for nervous problems, exhaustion, depression, emotional upsets, or debility following illness. The juice of fresh oats, pressed when still green, is similarly used as a nerve tonic.

Oatstraw baths are used in folk medicine to counter rheumatic pains. Make an infusion using 2 large handfuls of oatstraw with 2 quarts of water, strain and add this to the bath. Pillows filled with soothing and relaxing oatstraw have also been recommended for relieving insomnia.

As a home remedy oatmeal is excellent in skin washes for eczema and dry skin; add a tablespoon to a bowl of warm water and use for washing. Recent research suggests that oatbran (and to a lesser extent oatmeal) can also help to reduce blood cholesterol levels and should be regularly included in the diet of those at risk for heart disease or atherosclerosis.

Onion   *(Allium cepa)*

Like garlic, onion has long been used to combat infections, improve the digestion and ease coughs. Like garlic, the onion owes much of its smell to a number of sulphur compounds which stimulate the digestive system and have an antibiotic action, preventing decay.

Part used: Bulb.

Actions: Antibacterial, anti-inflammatory, cholagogue, diuretic, expectorant, hypotensive, lowers blood sugar.

Uses: In the home onions are ideal for coughs, catarrh, sore throats, sinusitis and fevers. Externally they can combat warts, insect stings, burns, cuts and boils. One of the most popular recipes for home-made cough syrup is simply to layer slices of onion with honey or sugar and leave overnight. In the morning a clear syrup can be collected which makes an effective, if not particularly pleasant-tasting, remedy for stubborn coughs.

Slices of raw onion can be applied directly to soothe insect stings (both bees and wasps) and can be used chopped in poultices for chilblains and to draw boils. Onion juice (made by pulping onions in a food processor) can be used to draw boils or to dab onto warts twice a day. It also makes a cleansing internal supplement to help maintain a healthy gut flora (important for those prone to candidiasis) and prevent fermentation. Take a tablespoon of the juice 3 times daily.

The heart of a cooled, boiled onion was once inserted into the ear to relieve earache, while a bowl of hot boiled onions with plenty of pepper was once standard fare for any threatening chill. Onion soup is ideal for colds and catarrh; drink 1-2 servings daily whenever you have a cold. The herb's cleansing action makes it a valuable addition to the diet for arthritics, gout sufferers or where fluid retention is a problem. Today, we also know that the onion will reduce both blood pressure and cholesterol levels, thus helping to combat any tendency for heart disease. Try to eat a serving of onions every day in soups, vegetable dishes, casseroles or salads.

Peppermint   (*Mentha X piperita*)

There are thought to be around 30 different species of mint, but since the plants readily cross-pollinate and hybridize no one is really certain. Peppermint is the variety most widely used in herbal medicine and is believed to be a cross between spearmint (*M. spicata*) and water mint (*M. aquatica*); it has a high menthol content, hence the characteristic smell. Spearmint is most often grown in gardens and makes an adequate substitute. It does not have the high menthol content of peppermint so is far less an irritant and therefore more suitable for children.

Description: A creeping perennial which can easily become invasive, with smooth lanceolate leaves and purple-tinged stems. Purple flowers are borne in long terminal spikes in the summer.

Part used: Leaves.

Actions: Analgesic, anti-emetic, antispasmodic, carminative, cholagogue, digestive tonic, peripheral vasodilator, diaphoretic but also cooling internally.

Uses: Mint is ideal to stimulate the digestion; drink a cup of peppermint or spearmint tea after meals (use 1 teaspoon to a cup of water) and is also warming and decongestant in colds and catarrh. Peppermint tea can also help to relieve nausea (including morning sickness).

An essential oil distilled from the leaves is antiseptic and mildly anesthetic. It can be used in stimulating rubs for rheumatism and bronchial congestion; put 5 drops in 1 tablespoon of almond oil and massage into aching muscles or the chest; 2 or 3 drops of peppermint oil in the bath can be especially restorative. To relieve nasal congestion put a couple of drops on a handkerchief and sniff it frequently. A drop on a cotton swab applied to the gum can also relieve toothache in neighboring teeth.

Caution: Peppermint should not be given to babies or toddlers in any form; excess of the oil can irritate the stomach lining, and misuse may lead to ulceration. The herb can also cause an allergic reaction in sensitive individuals.

Pineapple   (*Ananas sativa*)

Pineapple contains an enzyme called bromelain which acts as a digestive stimulant, making it ideal for easing indigestion and gastritis. This enzyme has a local action on the digestive tract but is not significantly absorbed into the system so does not affect the liver. The fruit is highly nutritious, rich in minerals and is a useful food for those prone to iron-deficient anemia or for debility and convalescence.

Part used: Fruit.

Actions: Anti-inflammatory, diuretic, digestive tonic, nutrient.

Uses: Drinking a glass of pineapple juice before meals can help stimulate a sluggish digestion; for the same reason it is sometimes used as a slimming aid. Externally, crushed pineapple can help to heal ulcers and slow-healing wounds, while the juice can also be used to tonify the skin. Gargling with the juice is a useful alternative for sore throats.

Plantain   (*Plantago* spp.)

Common plaintain (*P. major*) is a familiar garden weed often found filling the cracks in paved patios and dominating lawns. The plant has long been regarded as an important healing herb; Pliny even suggests that if several pieces of flesh are put in a pot with plantain, they will join back together again.

Description: Common plantain is characterized by its rat-tail like flower spikes and basal rosette of fleshy, rounded or ovate leaves. It grows to around 6 inches in height and is commonly found in gardens and pavement cracks. Ribwort plaintain (*P. lanceolata*) is taller, up to 24 inches, with more pointed, lance-shaped leaves with two to five prominent ribs. The flowers are dark rust with clear white feathery stamens and appear from May to September.

Part used: Leaves.

Actions: Common plantain is antibacterial, antihistamine, antiallergenic, astringent, blood tonic, demulcent, diuretic, expectorant, styptic; ribwort plantain is anticatarrhal, antispasmodic, relaxing expectorant and tonifies mucous membranes.

Uses: Externally the leaves make a good emergency treatment for irritant insect bites while, internally, common plantain tea (made from 2 teaspoons of dried leaves to a cup of water) can be helpful for gastric irritations, irritable bowel, hemorrhoids, cystitis or heavy periods. A tablespoon of plantain juice (made by pulping the leaves in a food processor) mixed with a teaspoon of honey, is a soothing remedy for cuts and minor wounds.

Common plantain's close relative, ribwort plantain, is more likely to be found in the hedgerow. An infusion (2 teaspoons of dried herb to a cup of water) can be used for colds, hay fever and allergic rhinitis. It contains minerals and trace elements. Particularly rich in zinc, potassium and silica, it can be helpful as a tissue healer and immune stimulant. Ribwort also contains aucubin, an antibiotic glycoside, which helps to make the plant very healing and supportive for the immune system.

Potato   (*Solanum tuberosum*)

Potatoes belong to the same family as deadly nightshade and henbane and, like these highly toxic herbs, contain poisonous alkaloids. Solanine, found in potato skin, has the same sort of antispasmodic properties as atropine (found in deadly nightshade) and in large quantities would be equally fatal. Indeed, if the potato were discovered today, the presence of such a potent alkaloid would probably mean that the scientists would condemn it as not safe for human consumption. Fortunately, potatoes were introduced into Western civilization in a more adventurous age; they were brought to Europe from Peru in 1530, but it took around 200 years for them to supplant bread, barley and carrots as a main dietary staple, partly because of the association with the nightshade family. Potatoes are an important source of vitamin C; they are also rich in B-complex vitamins (including B_1, B_5, B_6 and folic acid) and contain several minerals including iron, calcium, manganese, magnesium and phosphorus.

Part used: Tuber.

Actions: Antispasmodic, mild anodyne, digestive remedy, diuretic, emollient, nutrient.

Uses: In the days when every housewife knew how to make a poultice, mashed potato was the preferred choice of many and was widely applied to just about every ache, pain and inflammation. Besides being an important food source, potato juice is a useful addition to the medicine chest. It can be helpful for relieving digestive problems associated with excessive stomach acid including indigestion, gastritis and peptic ulcers, and is a good liver remedy which can be helpful for gall stones and other gallbladder problems. To collect the juice, thinly slice a raw potato and sprinkle with a very little salt. Leave in a shallow dish overnight and collect the resulting juices next morning. A little juice applied to the temples can relieve headaches.

Externally, slices of raw potato can be used to soothe skin inflammations, chilblains, burns and scalds (use grated raw potato mixed with a little vegetable oil to bind it). The same mix can soothe chapped and cracked skin.

Rosemary (*Rosmarinus officinalis*)

Rosemary is traditionally associated with remembrance; sprigs were exchanged by lovers or scattered on coffins. It is an apt association as rosemary has a stimulating effect on the nervous system and a reputation for improving the memory.

Description: An aromatic, evergreen shrub with tough, needle-like leaves and lilac to dark blue flowers in spring. Grows to six feet or more and will spread to a bushy plant six feet wide.

Parts used: Leaves, essential oil.

Actions: Leaves: antiseptic, antidepressive, antispasmodic, astringent, cardiac tonic, carminative, cholagogue, circulatory stimulant, diaphoretic, digestive remedy, diuretic, nervine, restorative tonic for nervous system; topical essential oil: analgesic, antirheumatic, rubefacient.

Uses: As a nerve tonic rosemary can be helpful for temporary fatigue and overwork; drink an infusion made with 1 heaped teaspoon of rosemary leaves to a cup of boiling water to relieve headaches, migraines, indigestion and coldness associated with poor circulation. It is a pleasant-tasting drink and, since rosemary is an evergreen, one that can be made using fresh herb throughout the year.

The essential oil made by steam-distilling the leaves is a valuable remedy for arthritis, rheumatism and muscular aches and pains. Use 10 drops of rosemary oil to a teaspoon of almond oil as a massage oil for aches and pain. A few drops added to the rinse water after shampooing will help clear dandruff and improve hair quality.

Sage   (*Salvia officinalis*)

Sage, an herb that is traditionally associated with longevity, is known to contain powerful antioxidants which can in fact combat cellular aging. It is also rich in estrogen so could almost be regarded as an early and very gentle form of hormone replacement therapy.

Description: An evergreen shrub, much branched, with velvety grey-green pointed leaves and flower spikes of blue or pink flowers in summer. Herbalists traditionally prefer the red sage (*S. officinalis pur-*

purescens group), which has red leaves, but both varieties are equally suitable for medicinal use.

Parts used: Leaves, essential oil.

Actions: Leaves: Antispasmodic, antiseptic, astringent, carminative, healing to mucosa, cholagogue, lowers blood sugar levels, peripheral vasodilator, suppresses perspiration, reduces salivation and lactation, uterine stimulant, systemically antibiotic; essential oil: antiseptic, antispasmodic, astringent, hypertensive, stimulant, emmenagogue, antioxidant.

Uses: Sage also dries up body fluids which, combined with its hormonal action, makes it ideal for relieving night sweats during menopause and for drying up milk in lactating mothers on weaning. The plant has an affinity with the throat and makes an excellent gargle and mouth wash for minor infections and inflammations. Use a standard infusion of 2 teaspoons of herb to a cup of water, and allow to cool before straining the mix and gargling. The same tea is ideal for indigestion. Drink a cup regularly as a tonic to combat the effects of old age.

In many parts of Europe, sage ointment is a favorite household standby for minor cuts and insect bites.

Siberian Ginseng (*Eleutherococcus senticosus*)

Siberian ginseng is a comparative newcomer to the West, rediscovered in the 1930s in Russia and then extensively used by Soviet athletes to increase stamina and enhance performance. It has been used in Chinese medicine for around 2,000 years and was traditionally regarded as a warming herb to strengthen the sinews and bones and improve energy and blood flow, especially in the elderly. Siberian ginseng has been extensively researched and is known to stimulate the immune and circulatory systems and also to help regulate blood pressure.

Part used: Root.

Actions: Adrenal stimulant, antiviral, adaptogen, aphrodisiac, combats the actions of stress, immune stimulant, lowers blood sugar levels, peripheral vasodilator, tonic.

Uses: Siberian ginseng is ideal for helping the body cope with stress; take up to 600 mg a day in capsules or tablets for 10 days before a busy work period, stressful exams or other additional strains. It can increase stamina and help the body cope more efficiently with both physical and mental stresses. As a home remedy Siberian ginseng is ideal to counter jet lag (see p. 108) and is an ideal all-round energy tonic for tiredness and fatigue.

Skullcap   *(Scutellaria lateriflora)*

Virginian skullcap is mainly used as a sedative and nervine by Western herbalists, but it can also be used to reduce fevers, calm the fetus and simulate digestion. Like all skullcaps, the plant takes its name from the dish-shaped seed pods.

Description: A spreading perennial with oval, toothed leaves and characteristic pink or blue tubular flowers to one side of the stem in summer.

Parts used: Aerial parts.

Actions: Antibacterial, antispasmodic, cooling, digestive stimulant, hypotensive, lowers cholesterol levels, relaxing and restorative nervine, styptic.

Use: Drink a cup of skullcap tea (1 heaped teaspoon to a cup of water) to encourage relaxation and combat anxiety and nervous tension. Skullcap tea can also be useful to soothe premenstrual tension and is helpful for nervous digestive problems. Drink up to 4 cups a day.

Slippery Elm   (*Ulmus rubra*)

The bark of the slippery or red elm was one of the most widely used of Native American medicines. The Ozark Indians took it for colds and bowel complaints while the Houmas used it for dysentery and the Missouri valley tribes used a decoction as a laxative. The bark is highly mucilaginous and provides a protective coating for the stomach. Thus it is ideal to soothe the mucous membranes in gastritis, ulceration and heartburn.

Part used: Bark.

Actions: Antitussive, cleansing, demulcent, expectorant, healing, nutrient; topically emollient.

Uses: As well as being extremely soothing and demulcent, slippery elm is also highly nutritious and is a useful dietary supplement in debility and convalescence. It is always sold powdered and can be made into a gruel by mixing ½ teaspoon with a little water to form a paste and then adding enough boiling water or milk to make up 1 cup. The gruel can be flavored with honey and a little cinnamon. The powder can also be added to hot cereal or muesli.

Slippery elm tablets are worth keeping in the household medicine chest as a useful remedy for indigestion and they can be taken before a journey to combat travel sickness. A couple of tablets taken before a party can also reduce the likelihood of a hangover as the stomach coating will help reduce alcohol absorption.

Externally slippery elm can be used to soothe wounds and burns and it is also commercially available in ointments (sometimes combined with marshmallow—*Althaea officinalis*) as a drawing remedy for splinters and boils.

St. John's Wort   (*Hypericum perforatum*)

St. John's wort is an extremely effective antidepressant which is believed to inhibit the enzyme monoamine oxidase (MAO), which itself inhibits neurotransmitters involved in stimulating the brain. MAO inhibitors are widely used in orthodox medicine, and some researchers suggest St. John's wort has similar action but without the usual side-effects of pharmaceutical drugs.

Description: An upright perennial growing from a woody base with linear ovate leaves which appear to be speckled with tiny holes when held to the light (they are, in fact, small oil sacs). The flowers are yellow with five petals and red-tipped stamens. It will grow to around 24 inches and flowers in midsummer.

Parts used: Flowering tops collected in midsummer, leaves collected before or after flowering.

Actions: Astringent, analgesic, anti-inflammatory, antidepressant, sedative, restorative tonic for the nervous system.

Uses: Externally, St. John's wort is one of our most useful first aid remedies. As an infused oil it can soothe minor burns, sunburns, cuts, scrapes and inflammations. It can soothe both skin and joint inflammations: add 2 drops of yarrow essential oil to a teaspoon of St. John's wort infused oil to make a helpful rub for tennis elbow.

Internally, St. John's wort tea acts as a tonic and restorative for the nervous system and, thanks to its analgesic effect, can also relieve menstrual pain and other abdominal aches. It has become extremely popular in Germany where it is widely prescribed by general practitioners as a safe, effective and nonaddictive alternative to orthodox antidepressants. Recent interest has also focussed on hypericins, found in the plant, which have a beneficial effect on the immune system and have been used in AIDS treatment. Drink a cup of St. John's wort tea (made by mixing 2 teaspoons of the dried flowering tops to a cup of water) for menstrual pain, insomnia and mild depression.

Caution: Prolonged use may increase the photosensitivity of the skin in sensitive individuals, although actual clinical reports of such incidences are extremely rare and the herb is regarded as safe in moderate use. Prolonged depression generally requires professional help; do not depend on self-help remedies.

Stinging Nettle (*Urtica dioica*)

Nettles sting because the hairs on their stems and leaves contain histamine, which is a potent skin irritant. Thanks to its ability to "rob the soil" and concentrate minerals and vitamins in its leaves, nettle is a good nutrient and makes a healthful spring tonic as well as a good supplement for iron-deficient anemia.

Description: A coarse perennial with ovate, toothed leaves covered with hairs. The flowers are small and green and hang in drooping clusters up to four inches long. The plant has creeping yellow roots and can be difficult to eradicate.

Parts used: Aerial parts, roots.

Actions: Antiseptic, antirheumatic, astringent, blood tonic, diuretic, expectorant, galactagogue, hypotensive, lowers blood sugar levels, important source of minerals, clears uric acid.

Uses: Nettles can be used externally in washes or hot infused oils for irritant skin rashes or as the base for massage rubs for rheumatism. Internally, nettle tea (made by adding 1 heaped teaspoon to a cup of boiling water) is also a popular folk remedy for rheumatism and can help to relieve the acute painful stage of gout. In pregnancy, nettle tea provides a useful additional source of calcium and iron and it also stimulates milk flow when breast-feeding. Nettle tea can also be helpful internally for allergic skin rashes, especially those connected with salicylate sensitivity (p. 88); drink up to 3 cups daily. The plant will also reduce blood sugar levels so is a useful addition to dietary control of adult-onset diabetes. Processing fresh young nettles in a juicer is a good way to make an energizing tonic; they can also be cooked in soups to help clear out the stagnations of winter. Simmer 3 cups of young nettle leaves with 3 cups of vegetable or chicken stock for 20 minutes, or until the nettles are tender; season well, and then blend in a food processor.

Tea   (*Camellia sinensis*)

When tea was first introduced into Europe in the 17th century it was regarded not as an everyday drink, but as a medicinal herb. Numerous tea house advertisements from the time extol the plants' virtues as a digestive remedy and cure for overindulgence. Tea has been drunk in China since around 3000 B.C. Most of the tea drunk in the West is black tea made by fermenting the leaves, while green tea is made from leaves that have been pan-fried and then dried. Oolong tea is a partly fermented variation.

Parts used: Leaves and leaf buds.

Actions: Stimulant, antibacterial, antioxidant, astringent, diuretic; some varieties reduce cholesterol levels and antitumor properties are reported in green teas.

Uses: The tea plant has a stimulating effect on the nervous system because of its caffeine-like alkaloids. Green tea is believed to improve resistance to stomach and skin cancers and stimulate the immune system, while oolong tea is generally regarded as a digestive remedy which it is now known can reduce cholesterol levels. Thus it may be useful to combat arteriosclerosis. In China, green tea is considered cooling and is preferred in hot weather, while oolong and black teas are more warming for cold days.

Black tea is especially astringent and is ideal (unsweetened and without milk) to ease diarrhea. It is also a traditional Cantonese remedy for hangovers. Green tea is especially rich in fluoride, so it can help combat any tendency for tooth decay. It is also useful to soothe insect bites: apply either damp green tea leaves or an infused green tea bag directly onto the affected area. Green tea is also reputed to have antiviral activity, so it can be helpful to drink four or five cups a day when suffering from colds or influenza.

Tea Tree   (*Melaleuca alternifolia*)

Extracts from the Australian tea tree were originally used by the Aborigines as a wound remedy. By the Second World War it was a regular component in field dressing kits among Australian troops. The plant was first studied in Europe in the 1920s when French researchers found that tea tree oil, collected by steam distillation, was a more effective antiseptic than phenol and had impressive antibiotic properties. In the past few years a thriving tea tree industry has grown up which has led to a number of highly adulterated oils appearing on the market. True tea tree oil is one of the few oils that does not usually irritate mucous membranes and it can be used undiluted on the skin.

Part used: Essential oil.

Actions: Antibacterial, antifungal, antiseptic, antiviral, diaphoretic, expectorant.

Uses: Tea tree is ideal externally for any sort of infection. Both the oil and cream are widely available and can be used as a wound dressing or to treat fungal problems like yeast infections or athlete's foot. The herb is also a useful expectorant and is sometimes found in over-the-counter cough lozenges. It can also be used on a tampon to treat vaginal yeast infections (see p. 101).

Tea tree is helpful for acne and other minor skin problems; make a lotion by adding 40 drops of tea tree oil to ½ cup of rosewater and ½ cup of distilled witch hazel. Store in a dark glass bottle and shake well before use. Apply with a cotton swab 3 or 4 times a day.

A drop of tea tree oil, applied undiluted, can help prevent cold sores developing if used as soon as the pricking sensation that heralds the sore starts, or it can help soothe them once they appear. It is also effective on warts. Use one drop each morning directly on the wart. Tea tree cream can be used to soothe insect bites and tea tree diluted in water (20 drops in one cup of water) can be used in a spray as an insect repellent. The oil, used undiluted on a comb or added to shampoos (10 drops to 1 tablespoon of shampoo), can be used for head lice and nits in children.

Thyme (*Thymus vulgaris*)

Like many culinary herbs, thyme is a soothing digestive remedy which can stimulate the digestion as it copes with rich foods. The plant (particularly the oil) is also extremely antiseptic, and is a good expectorant, helping both to clear phlegm and, thanks to its antibacterial action, combat chest infections.

Description: A low-growing, variable perennial shrub with small pointed grey-green leaves and white to purple flowers in summer.

Parts used: Aerial parts, essential oil.

Actions: Antibiotic, antiseptic, antispasmodic, antimicrobial, antitussive, astringent, carminative, diuretic, expectorant, wound herb; topically rubefacient.

Uses: As an antiseptic expectorant, common thyme is useful in cough syrups and combines well with licorice. Make a cough syrup by combining the infusion (1 teaspoon to a cup) with honey (see p. 55) or drink thyme tea as a tonic for exhaustion or to regulate the digestion. The fresh leaves can be crushed and applied to minor wounds and warts.

Thyme oil is used in aromatherapy for muscular aches, pains and stiffness or can be added to baths to combat exhaustion. Use 10 drops of oil in 1 teaspoon of almond oil and massage gently into aching limbs.

Witch Hazel   (*Hamamelis virginiana*)

The witch hazel tree was used for numerous ills by several Native American tribes especially for back and muscle aches. Today, the bark is steam-distilled to produce the familiar clear, "distilled witch hazel" available from any pharmacy.

Part used: Bark.

Actions: Astringent, anti-inflammatory, styptic.

Uses: Distilled witch hazel is an essential in the first aid kit; it can heal bruises, sprains, nosebleeds, cuts and scrapes, spots and blemishes, and can ease the pain of varicose veins and hemorrhoids. Press a cotton swab soaked in witch hazel to cuts to stop bleeding or insert a swab into a nostril for nosebleeds. Use a witch hazel compress for sprains and bruises.

Taken internally, an infusion of the leaves (1 teaspoon of chopped leaves to a cup of water) is effective for treating diarrhea, colitis and heavy periods.

Yarrow (*Achillea millefolium*)

A common meadow herb, yarrow's botanical name is derived from the Greek hero Achilles, who reputedly used the plant as a wound herb during the Trojan wars. The plant was once used in divination, and folk rituals still associate it with prediction (generally for identifying future husbands); the same tradition persists in China, where yarrow stalks are used with the *I Ching*.

Description: A perennial herb with distinctive feathery leaves and tiny white flowers in clusters appearing throughout the summer and autumn.

Parts used: Leaves collected throughout the growing season, flowers gathered when in full bloom.

Actions: Anti-inflammatory, antispasmodic, astringent, bitter, carminative, diaphoretic, digestive tonic, diuretic, febrifuge, hypotensive, peripheral vasodilator, styptic, urinary antiseptic.

Uses: One of yarrow's country names is nosebleed, which confirms its traditional first aid use as an emergency styptic; simply insert a couple of fresh leaves into the nostril, and the feathery leaves provide an ideal encouragement for clotting.

Yarrow relaxes the peripheral blood vessels and thus can help to reduce high blood pressure; it is also cooling in fevers. Yarrow tea can be helpful for colds, influenza, hay fever and catarrh, and it can also be added to urinary remedies. Use 1 heaped teaspoon of herb to a cup of boiling water and drink up to 3 cups daily for catarrhal problems or colds.

Like chamomile, yarrow flowers also contain antiallergenic compounds which are activated by steam so are only found in infusions or the distilled essential oil. These compounds make yarrow ideal for steam inhalations for hay fever or allergic rhinitis.

Yarrow oil is available commercially and is also antiinflammatory. It can be used in chest rubs for colds and catarrh (use 2 drops to a teaspoon of sweet almond oil) and is also helpful for tennis elbow and joint inflammations when combined with St. John's wort infused oil (see p. 56).

Caution: Yarrow should be avoided in pregnancy as it is a uterine stimulant. The fresh herb can sometimes cause contact dermatitis and, in rare cases, prolonged use may increase the skin's photosensitivity.

How to Prepare Herbal Medicines

Making your own herbal remedies is no more difficult than blending sauces or cooking vegetables. Basic kitchen equipment is all that is needed, although if remedies are to be kept for any length of time, it is important to use sterile bottles and jars for storage.

This section details simple methods for making the sorts of remedies needed to deal with minor ailments and first aid in the home. Creams, ointments, pessaries, capsules and tinctures are available ready-made from health food stores and pharmacies.

INFUSIONS

An infusion is simply a tea made by steeping an herb in freshly boiled water for 10 minutes; it is an ideal method for most leafy herbs and flowers. Typically use 1 to 2 teaspoons of herb to a cup of water (1 cup = 8 fluid ounces). The herb needs to be put into a ceramic or glass teapot, jug or cup (with lid). It is important for the water to go just off the boil, otherwise many aromatic plant constituents will be lost in the excessive steam. After infusing, strain through a sieve and take a cup three times a day. Sweeten with a little honey if desired.

If using fresh herb you need three times as much herb to allow for the additional weight of water in fresh plant material, i.e. 1-2 tablespoons per cup of water. An infusion can be reheated before each dose but it is best to make only enough infusion for one dose or one day's dosages at a time even though surplus can be stored in the refrigerator for up to 48 hours.

DECOCTIONS

A decoction is a tea made by simmering the plant material for 15-20 minutes. It is ideal for tougher plant components such as barks, roots and berries, from which it can be more difficult to extract the active ingredients. Use 1 to 2 teaspoons of herb to 1½ cups of cold water which should then be brought to the boil in a stainless steel, glass, ceramic or enamel saucepan (not aluminum) and allowed to simmer until the volume has been reduced by about a third.

The mixture is then treated as an infusion: strained through a sieve and taken in cup doses during the day. Decoctions can be reduced after straining to between 1 to 2 tablespoons with further gentle heating. Then this concentrated mix can be used in drop dosages either as is or in water. This can be an effective way to administer decoctions to children who are often reluctant to drink whole cups of herbal brews.

COMBINED INFUSIONS AND DECOCTIONS

When using a number of herbs in a tea it is often necessary to use some as infusions and some as decoctions; for example, a tea of ginger root with elder flowers and yarrow for a cold. In these cases it is best to measure out the required 1½ cups of water (or 4½ cups if making enough for the day) and use this to simmer the required amount of ginger root (usually ½-1 teaspoon per dose). Once the volume has reduced by about a third, pour the still simmering mixture over the dried leaves and flowers, in a jug or cup, and infuse for another 10 to 15 minutes.

The tea can then be used in the same way as simple infusions or decoctions (see above).

SYRUPS

Sugar or honey can be used to preserve herbal infusions and decoctions and are ideal for cough remedies, as the sweetness is also soothing.

Syrups are easy to produce at home by using a standard infusion or decoction (depending on the type of herb to be used). After straining the mixture, make a syrup by adding 3 cups of liquid to 1 cup of unrefined sugar or honey. Heat the mixture in a cast iron or stainless steel saucepan, stirring constantly to dissolve the sugar or honey and make the syrup. Allow the mixture to cool and store in clean glass bottles with a cork, not a screw-top. Using a cork is important as syrups often ferment, and tight screw-tops can easily cause bottles to explode.

STEAM INHALANTS

Inhaling aromatic oils is a good way to clear the respiratory system of mucus in catarrhal conditions. Both infusions and well-diluted essential oils can be used, although it is important to stay in a warm room for 30 minutes after treatment to allow the airways time to return to normal.

Use around 1 pint of a standard infusion or add up to 10 drops of essential oil to a bowl of hot water per treatment. Useful inhalant herbs include chamomile, thyme, eucalyptus and peppermint. Repeat treatments once or twice a day inhaling the steam for 10 minutes each time.

FOOTBATHS

Soaking your feet in a hot bath can bring much needed relief to aching feet, ease sprains, stimulate the circulation for those prone to chilblains and also help to combat the common cold. Suitable essential oils or hot infusions can be used or one can opt for a traditional mustard bath (see p. 33). Alternating hot and cold treatments can help reduce bruising and provide emergency relief for badly sprained ankles. Soak the feet or other affected area in a basin of very hot water containing a large amount of rosemary sprigs or 20 drops of rosemary essential oil for 3 to 5 minutes and then plunge into a water and ice mixture for 2 to 3 minutes. Repeat the process for as long as you can bear.

INFUSED OILS

Infused oils can be used as a base for massage and chest rubs. There are two techniques: hot infusion and cold infusion.

Hot infused oils: These are made by heating 2 cups of dried herb in 1 pint of sunflower (or similar) oil in a double boiler over water for about three hours. Remember to refill the lower saucepan with hot water from time to time to prevent it from boiling dry. After about three hours the oil will take on a greenish color and it can then be strained and squeezed through a muslin bag and stored in clean glass bottles, away from direct sunlight. This method is suitable for making comfrey, chickweed, stinging nettle or infused rosemary oil.

Cold infused oils: Because the oil is not heated in this method, you can use good quality seed oils that are rich in essential fatty acids (EFAs) which have significant therapeutic properties. Oils high in EFAs include walnut, safflower and pumpkin oils. The cold infused oil is made by simply filling a large screw-top jar (such as a clean instant coffee jar) with the dried or fresh herb and then completely covering with oil. The jar should be left on a sunny windowsill for at least three weeks. Then the mixture can be strained through a muslin bag. The cold infused method is suitable for St. John's wort, marigold or chamomile flowers.

MASSAGE OILS

The sort of massage oils used in aromatherapy are very easy to make at home by adding a few drops of essential oil to some sort of oil base. Suitable bases include sweet almond oil, wheat germ oil, avocado oil or any of the infused herb oils made from walnut or sunflower oil described above.

In general do not use more than 10 percent of essential oil (10 drops of essential oil in a teaspoon of carrier oil) as many essential oils can irritate sensitive skins. Always buy good quality organically grown essential oils as many cheaper ones are chemically adulterated or contain pollutants.

COMPRESSES

Compresses are often used to accelerate the healing of wounds or muscle injuries. They are basically cloth pads soaked in herbal extracts and usually applied hot to painful limbs, swellings or strains. Use a clean piece of cotton, flannel, linen or surgical gauze soaked in a hot, strained infusion, decoction or tincture (diluted with hot water) and apply to the affected area. When the compress cools, repeat using fresh, hot mixture.

Occasionally a cold compress may be used, as with some types of headaches when a cool pad soaked in lavender infusion can be helpful.

POULTICES

Poultices have a very similar action to compresses but involve directly applying the whole herb to an affected area rather than using a liquid extract. Poultices are usually applied hot for swellings, sprains or to draw pus or splinters. As with hot compresses, renew the hot poultice as it cools or place a hot water bottle on top to keep it hot.

To make a poultice, simply bruise fresh herbs—mix in a food processor for a few seconds or sweat them in a pan— then spread the mixture onto gauze and apply to the affected area. Dried herbs or powders need to first be mixed with hot water to form a paste; then squeeze out any surplus liquid and spread the residue on gauze or apply directly to the area affected. Alternatively, mix the herb powders with mashed potato and use that as a poultice.

If putting poultices directly to the skin, apply a little vegetable oil first to prevent it from sticking too much.

BUYING AND STORING HERBS

Always buy herbs in small quantities (½ to 1 pound at a time) to avoid unnecessary home storage. Where possible, examine material before buying to check on quality. Choose herbs which have a good color and aroma and are not faded or musty smelling. Avoid shops which display herbs in clear glass jars on sunny shelves; the quality will probably be poor. Inadequate storage can lead to rapid deterioration with mouse droppings, mold and insects among unwanted pollutants.

Ideally, buy organic herbs or those labeled as "wild crafted" which means they have been collected in the wild rather than grown as a commercial (and often heavily sprayed) cash crop. Poor harvesting can lead to many unwanted additions—dried grass, for example, is often found with herbs like eyebright, which have been gathered from meadow areas. With practice one can soon recognize the characteristics of many dried herbs so it becomes easier to check on the accuracy of labels. Skullcap, for example, has characteristic seed pods, and many herbs can be identified from their aroma.

Mistakes can and do happen, however. One well-documented error concerned the supplier who sold sea mayweed (*Matricaria maritima*) as feverfew. The plants are similar in appearance, but the mayweed lacks feverfew's therapeutic chemicals and is useless for treating migraine.

Herbs For Common Ailments

This section lists those common ailments that may require emergency treatment as well as disorders that are self-limiting and would normally be treated at home with over-the-counter medicines.

In all cases, if symptoms persist for more than a couple of days or if the condition appears to worsen, seek medical help immediately.

Note: In general "oil" refers to the essential oil; use of an infused oil is always specified as such. Herbal quantities in teas are for dried herbs. Refer to the specific herbs described in the previous chapter for cautions on individual herbs. Unless otherwise specified, doses should be repeated up to 3 times a day.

ACNE AND BLEMISHES

The characteristic pimples and blackheads of acne are all too familiar to teenagers. The cause of the problem is usually inflamed sebaceous glands which open into the hair follicles and produce an oil secretion known as sebum. This oil helps to keep the skin soft, moist and supple. The sebaceous glands are at their most active during puberty, and it is a time when the excess oils can block skin pores and lead to bacterial infection with pus-filled pimples, small cysts and blackheads. Typically, acne starts in the early teens and usually disappears by the mid-20s, although a tendency to blemishes can be a lifelong problem for some people.

Cutting down on the foods which might encourage sebaceous gland activity—refined carbohydrates (typically sugar and white flour), fried foods and animal fats—is important. Sweets and chocolates also tend to aggravate the condition as do alcohol and sweet, sugary drinks.

Infected pustules will generally respond to low doses of echinacea (1 200-mg capsule 2 to 3 times daily) or use echinacea creams externally.

Cleansing Tea for Acne

2 parts stinging nettle
1 part each chamomile and marigold flowers

Mix the herbs and use two teaspoons of the mix to a cup of boiling water. Drink a cup 3 times daily.

Another useful herb for acne, and one that can generally be found from North American suppliers, is gotu kola (*Centella asiatica*). Drink a tea made from 1 heaped teaspoon of the dried herb to a cup of water 3 times a day.

Externally, the classic treatment is to rub acne pustules with a cut garlic clove, an effective remedy, but not one that teenage sufferers enthusiastically embrace! Alternatively try cabbage lotion (p. 78) or the following mixture of essential oils in an astringent base:

Cleansing Lotion for Acne

5 drops each of tea tree, eucalyptus and lavender oils
2 Tbsp. each of distilled witch hazel and water

Mix together and store in a clean glass bottle. Shake
the bottle well before applying to affected areas
night and morning with a cotton swab.

ATHLETE'S FOOT

Athlete's foot (*Tinea pedis*) is a very common fungal
infection generally affecting the space between the toes
and toe nails. Depending on the infecting fungus it can
either include inflammation and itching or may simply
involve scaling of the skin and general discomfort. Like
all their species, the yeasts causing athlete's foot thrive
in warm, damp places, so good sensible foot care (making sure the toes are well dried after bathing and that
shoes are comfortable) is important.

Antifungal creams, such as marigold and echinacea,
can help. Apply them night and morning to affected
areas. Alternatively soak the feet at night in a footbath
containing a marigold infusion made from 1 tablespoon
of petals to 1 quart of boiling water and allowed to
cool. Dry thoroughly afterwards.

BACKACHE

Backache is one of the most common causes of both
absence from work and seeking alternative medical

treatment. Thorough professional investigation is needed to identify the cause of the problem; this can range from pulled muscles and damaged discs to poor posture, kidney disease, gynecological problems or simply sitting in an awkward position for long periods.

Some sorts of backache are given rather grander labels. "Lumbago" simply means pain in the lower back (the lumbar region). "Sciatica" is a pain felt along the back and outer side of the thigh, leg and foot, with accompanying back pain and stiffness generally caused by a damaged disc putting pressure on either the sciatic nerve or one of the many other nerves which start in the lower back area. "Fibrositis" is an inflammation of fibrous tissue, especially muscle sheaths, which often affects the back muscles, leading to pain and stiffness.

Obviously all these different sorts of backache require very different treatments, so accurate diagnosis is important. Similarly if the cause is associated with kidney weakness or a displaced womb then these underlying causes need to be tackled as simple backache remedies will only provide symptomatic relief. In all these cases, professional advice is essential.

If the problem is really originating from the back itself then often treatment from an osteopath, chiropractor or acupuncturist can solve the problem. Massage from a therapeutic masseur or physiotherapist can also give relief, while poor posture can be corrected by learning the Alexander Technique.

For persistent backache with no obvious cause, changing sleeping positions can sometimes help. A firm, supportive mattress is essential. Lying on your back with knees bent and curling into a small ball with the spine curved can often bring relief.

A relaxing soak in a hot bath can also help. Add up to 5 drops of essential oils of eucalyptus, juniper, lavender, rosemary or thyme to the bath water. Massage rubs are also helpful, especially if you have a friend or partner who can help with the massage.

Massage Oil for Backache

- 10 drops each of lavender, eucalyptus and thyme essential oils
- 5 drops juniper essential oil
- 2 tablespoons of infused St. John's wort oil or infused comfrey oil

Mix all the oils together and store in a small dark glass bottle. Shake well before use and massage about ½ teaspoon of oil into the affected areas night and morning. If you do not have the infused oils, use almond or wheatgerm oil instead.

BOILS AND CARBUNCLES

A boil is a tender inflamed area of skin containing pus which is generally caused by a staphylococcal infection of a hair follicle or a break in the skin. A cluster of boils is known as a carbuncle.

Boils are usually a sign of reduced resistance to infection, perhaps because of general debility, chronic illness, exhaustion or overwork. There could also be some deep-seated septic focus, such as a dental abscess, adding to the overall toxicity. Frequent outbreaks of boils can suggest a more serious underlying cause, possibly diabetes or kidney disease.

Traditionally, poultices or drawing ointments are used to encourage the boil to discharge. Use commercially available slippery elm or chickweed ointments or a home-made hot infused oil of either herb. Alternatively make a slippery elm poultice by mixing a teaspoon of the powdered herb with just enough hot water or hot marigold infusion to make a thick paste. Apply this to the boil. Follow the instructions on p. 58 for applying poultices. Echinacea cream is also effective: apply the cream and cover with a Band-Aid.

Combine external treatment with herbs taken internally to boost the immune system and combat bacterial infections; take 2 200-mg capsules of either garlic or echinacea 2 times a day or add plenty of garlic to your cooking.

BRUISES

A bruise is an area of skin discoloration caused by blood escaping from damaged underlying blood vessels following injury; the familiar multicolored healing process occurs as the hemoglobin in the escaped blood breaks down into other chemicals before being completely dispersed.

A tendency to bruise easily can be related to problems with the blood's ability to clot or may simply suggest that small blood vessels are comparatively thin and easily damaged. This is often the case in otherwise fit and healthy women. If you do have blood which does not clot readily—or are on blood-thinning drugs—then avoid taking herbs like feverfew which can slow down clotting even further.

An ice pack in the form of a package of frozen peas provides an ideal emergency treatment to relieve the pain of a new bruise; alternating that with a hot water bottle can help to encourage reabsorption of blood and bring more rapid relief. Dabbing a little distilled witch hazel on the bruise is ideal or freeze the liquid in an ice-cube tray in the freezer and then simply rub a cube on the affected area.

Commercially available arnica or comfrey creams applied to unbroken skin will also encourage healing (or use home-made comfrey infused oil). If the bruise is the result of some traumatic accident, give homeopathic arnica 6x internally to calm the sufferer and encourage more rapid healing.

BUNIONS

These painful swellings of the joint between the big toe and the adjoining bone can be caused by badly fitting shoes, although a tendency to them can be hereditary. Ensuring that shoes are large and comfortable enough is essential; wear loose slippers or sandals at home. St. John's wort oil or cream applied regularly can be helpful or, if the bunion becomes particularly blistered and infected, use marigold cream at night. Long-term comfrey cream applied night and morning can help to repair damaged tissues, although it should not be used on broken skin.

BURNS AND SCALDS

Burns are potential medical emergencies and only the most minor should be treated at home. Any burn more than about 2 inches across should be seen by a doctor as soon as possible.

For less severe burns, run cold water over the affected area or use an ice pack (or package of frozen peas) to cool it down and ease the immediate pain. Keep the injury cool for two or three hours; use a clean cloth soaked in cold water, chilled marigold infusion (p. 31) or diluted lavender oil (combine a teaspoon of oil with a tablespoon of iced water) to cover the affected area. Fresh aloe vera gel is very cooling; if you have a plant, slit open a leaf and apply it to the burn after initially cooling with cold water. Infused St. John's wort oil is also ideal for minor burns; apply a little directly to the area after it has been kept cool for a couple of hours or use chickweed cream or infused oil in the same way.

For minor burns and scalds, slices of fresh cucumber, a purée of fresh cranberries (or cranberry juice), or a little grated raw potato can all be applied directly to the affected area and held in place with gauze and adhesive tape.

CATARRH AND SINUS PROBLEMS

Catarrh can take many forms—from thick mucus that makes breathing difficult to watery secretions causing a semipermanent drip; it has many different causes.

Catarrh can be a symptom of the common cold or it can be a sign of allergic reaction as in hay fever (p. 82); it can stay in the upper respiratory tract causing nasal congestion or affect the lower airways and be coughed up as phlegm. Lingering catarrh makes an ideal breeding ground for bacteria and can lead to inflammation of the sinuses.

Whatever the cause, diet is extremely important and,

as in the common cold, foods that encourage mucus formation should be avoided. These include refined carbohydrates, dairy products and alcohol. A fruit fast (three pieces of fruit at each meal and plenty of fruit juice) for 24 hours can help, while zinc and vitamin C supplements are useful to strengthen the immune system and combat infection.

Home self-help remedies for catarrh can include steam inhalations and teas. A useful inhalant can be made by putting 5 drops of thyme or eucalyptus oil in a basin containing a quart of boiling water (see p. 55). Alternatively use thyme or peppermint infusion as the inhalant, with 1 tablespoon of dried herb to 1 quart of boiling water.

Anti-catarrhal Tea

2 parts each of elderflower and yarrow
1 part each of thyme and ribwort plantain

Mix the dried herbs and use 2 tablespoons to 1 quart of boiling water. Drink a cup of the mixture 3 to 4 times daily.

Onion is very anticatarrhal so eat plenty of onion soup or a serving of hot boiled onions once a day.

CHILBLAINS

Chilblains are caused by a limited blood flow to the remoter parts of the body, generally in response to cold. In order to maintain vital organs and deep tissues at a suitably warm temperature, the blood flow to the fingers and toes is constricted. This leads to numbness, and the tissues become more alkaline because of the reduced levels of oxygen reaching them. When the temperature rises and blood supply returns, normal balance is restored and the familiar burning and itching sensation of chilblains follows.

Wearing adequate clothing on cold days is the easiest way to avoid occasional chilblains, while habitual sufferers can improve their circulation with teas of stimulating herbs like cinnamon and ginger (see p. 11). Using external creams and oils which encourage blood flow to a particular area may also be helpful for chronic sufferers. Massage the infused oils of cayenne or rosemary regularly into the toes or fingers prone to chilblains or use a mustard footbath (p. 33).

Arnica cream can help relieve the discomfort of chilblains once they've appeared but it should not be used on broken skin. Other helpful remedies to relieve symptoms include aloe vera gel or marigold cream. If nothing else is available, a poultice of grated raw onion or raw potato can ease the discomfort.

COLD SORES

Cold sores are caused by the herpes simplex virus which is believed to be carried by around 50 percent of the adult population. The sores are always quite localized and take the form of tiny blisters which usually start with a tingling sensation and rapidly develop into inflamed, red areas generally occurring around the mouth but sometimes found elsewhere on the body.

Once a person has been infected, the virus can remain dormant in the body for years, usually erupting whenever the sufferer is run-down or overtired. In women, the sores will often coincide with menstruation, and they also—as the name implies—tend to herald a cold or flu. The virus is extremely contagious during the blistering stage and can spread in saliva or by contact; however, cold sores are more of a nuisance than serious health hazard.

Useful herbal remedies include tea tree and lavender oils. Either put one drop of tea tree oil or tea tree cream directly on the sore as soon as the characteristic tingling sensation starts, or dilute 20 drops of lavender oil with 1 teaspoon of water and apply that using a cotton swab. Infused marigold oil can be used in the same way. If cold sores are a recurrent problem, take echinacea capsules (2 200-mg capsules 3 times a day) or drink 2 to 3 cups of echinacea tea (make a decoction using 2 teaspoons of root to 1½ cups of water) daily. Eat plenty of garlic and take a 1,000 mg tablet of vitamin C daily to strengthen the immune system and combat infection.

COLDS AND FLU

Colds can be caused by any one of hundreds of different viruses which can only survive in the body's cells and are usually passed from one person to another in droplets of moisture spread by coughs and sneezes. The viruses are constantly changing as they spread, so just because someone has caught a cold that is "going around" once, any immunity to that particular virus will be of little use if there is repeated infection. This is because the virus will have mutated into another form.

The herbal approach to treatment focuses on strengthening the body's immune system, thus helping it to fight the virus, while relieving symptoms. Frequent colds can be a sign of a weakened immunity; they can also indicate a stressful lifestyle or poor diet, and medicine alone can't help in these situations. Combating a cold at the first sign of symptoms is also important. Rather than trying to ignore the increasing catarrh and sore throat until the cold is full blown, start treatment immediately.

Echinacea is one of the best herbs to take to strengthen the immune system; also add plenty of garlic cloves in cooking. Anticatarrhals such as elderflower and yarrow can also ease symptoms. Cut down on refined carbohydrates (white sugar and white flour products) as these tend to encourage mucus, and eat plenty of fruit instead. Taking up to 5 g of vitamin C a day in divided doses can also help.

Tea for Colds

3 parts echinacea (preferably aerial parts of *E. purpurea* or use the root of any species—see p. 16)
2 parts each elderflower and yarrow
1 part each peppermint and thyme

Mix the elderflower, yarrow, thyme and peppermint—and the echinacea if using aerial parts—and make an infusion using 2 teaspoons of the mixture to a cup of water. If you have echinacea root then follow the instructions for a combination infusion/decoction (p. 54). Make a decoction of echinacea using 1 teaspoon of root to 1½ cups of boiling water. Pour this over 1 teaspoon of the herbal mixture above.

For aches and pains associated with the flu make the following infusion:

2 parts each dried echinacea leaves and boneset
1 part peppermint

Mix the herbs and use 2 teaspoons to 1 cup of water. Drink a cup 3 to 4 times a day while symptoms persist.

COUGHS

Coughing is the body's natural response to any blockage of the airways such as dust, traffic fumes or mucus resulting from infection. Coughing can also be a symptom of more serious illness, so professional medical attention is needed for any cough which persists for more than a few days or where there is no obvious cause.

Coughs can be dry and irritating or "productive" with phlegm which can vary in shade from white to green. Colored phlegm generally indicates an infection and, if it is streaked with blood then, professional medical help is needed. Dry coughs can often linger for weeks following a cold and in some cases can be a nervous habit.

Tea for Productive Coughs

3 parts thyme
2 parts licorice
1 part each elderflower, common plantain and fennel seed
Juice of ½ lemon per cup
Honey

Mix the thyme, elderflower, plantain and fennel

seeds. Make a combination infusion/decoction (p. 54) using 2 teaspoons of the licorice to 1½ quarts of water and then pour this over 1½ tablespoons of the dried herb mixture. Take a cup of the tea 3 times a day, reheating and adding the lemon juice and a teaspoon of honey before drinking.

If there is a lot of phlegm, eat at least 2 cloves of garlic a day; crush them, mix with a vinaigrette dressing and pour over a serving of lettuce leaves.

Chest rubs can also help to loosen phlegm. Mix 10 drops each of thyme and eucalyptus oil with a teaspoon of almond oil and rub well into the chest (front and back) night and morning. For congestion in babies and toddlers, put 2 to 3 drops of these oils onto a pillow or bib so that the child will gently inhale them.

CRAMPS

The severe pain of a cramp is caused by a sudden contraction of the muscles. Commonly this occurs in calf muscles which become hard and tense; rubbing the area vigorously can bring rapid relief. A cramp can also be caused by unusual exercise, stress, tiredness or poor posture or there might be an imbalance of the salts in the body.

In hot weather, cramps are often due to a shortage of salt related to dehydration so in hot climates taking salt tablets can be useful for those prone to cramps. Taking supplements of magnesium and vitamin B-complex can also help.

A massage rub containing 5 drops each of ginger, thyme and lavender oil in 1 tablespoon of almond oil can bring relief. If night cramps in the legs are a recurrent problem try massaging them with this mixture before going to bed, and seek professional help if the condition persists.

CUTS AND SCRAPES

Always bathe cuts and scrapes before applying antiseptic creams by either rinsing the wound under running water or using a cotton ball soaked in warm water, taking care to wipe from center to edge of the scrape to clear any grime. Infusions of antiseptic herbs, such as marigold, make a good wash instead of water. Press a clean tissue or gauze pad, ideally soaked in distilled witch hazel, over the injury for a few minutes to stop bleeding. Finally, apply an antiseptic cream.

There are many over-the-counter herbal products now available including marigold (*calendula*), echinacea, St. John's wort or tea tree creams which are all suitable and can be used on open wounds. Aloe vera creams can also be used on scrapes, and there are also various combinations of St. John's wort and marigold commercially available. Lemon balm cream can be helpful for wounds which are slow to heal. If a yarrow plant is handy, make a poultice using yarrow leaves (first rinsed in clean water if available) and press that to the affected area.

DIAPER RASH

No matter how frequently babies are changed and dried, most develop a red or sore bottom at some stage.

Keeping the affected area as dry as possible (even by blowing with a hair dryer set to the cool setting) is essential. Ointments are better to use than creams as they form a protective barrier for the skin, whereas creams tend to soak in and soften. Marigold or chamomile ointment can be helpful and safe to use, as can aloe vera gel. Comfrey ointment is especially healing, although some parents may prefer to avoid use of this herb because of reports of its toxicity (p. 14). Bacteria in the feces can react with urine to produce ammonia and this can encourage fungal infections to develop, similar to vaginal yeast infection. These are best treated with ointments containing marigold or tea tree applied after each change.

DIARRHEA

Causes of diarrhea can range from food poisoning and overeating to stress and anxiety. Diarrhea can also be a symptom of more serious disease, so persistent or recurrent diarrhea needs professional attention.

Sudden diarrhea is often caused by some sort of gastrointestinal infection or food poisoning (especially if others who shared the same meal are similarly affected) when there are also symptoms of nausea or vomiting. It is a common problem when visiting exotic locations (see p. 105), but it is the body's natural reaction to an infecting organism and is often the best way of getting rid of it quickly. Trying to stop the diarrhea can often cause more harm than good, and it is better simply to soothe the digestive tract with astringent herbs and let nature take its course. Strong cold Indian tea is rich in tannins and can ease an excessively overworked gut if nothing better is available; drink it without milk or sugar and add lemon juice and a pinch of cinnamon to ease the digestive tract and combat infection. You can eat raw, grated underripe apples and stewed cranberries or bilberries. A helpful herbal brew for diarrhea due to infection and gastroenteritis follows:

Tummy Tea

1 part each marigold petals and peppermint
2 parts meadowsweet

Mix the herbs together and use 1 teaspoon to a cup of boiling water; drink 1 cup every 2 to 3 hours.

Severe diarrhea depletes body fluids, so drink plenty of liquids; this is especially important in children and when the diarrhea is accompanied by vomiting. Carrot juice is also especially helpful for combating diarrhea. Take 2 200-mg echinacea capsules up to 3 times a day while symptoms last to counter infection. Slippery elm gruel (p. 44) will help to soothe inflammation in the gut as well as provide necessary nutrients; drink a cup 3 times a day.

Gastric flu and stomach chills can also lead to diarrhea. Again symptoms are likely to be short-lived; using these same astringent teas, combined with anti-infection herbs like echinacea and garlic, can help.

Regular diarrhea can often be stress-related; in severe cases it can take the form of ulcerative colitis, which needs professional treatment. The sort of increased frequency and loose stools which are so common before exams or job interviews can be soothed by chamomile tea (1 teaspoon to a cup of water).

Tea for Nervous Diarrhea

3 parts meadowsweet
2 parts lemon balm
1 part skullcap

Mix the herbs and use 2 teaspoons to a cup of boiling water. Drink up to 3 cups a day.

EARACHE

Earache can be an extremely painful and distressing condition, especially in children, and needs great care in home treatment as infection can lead to perforated ear drums and the risk of permanent hearing damage. The cause is usually an acute local infection, which can be related to sinus or catarrhal problems; the anticatarrhal tea and steam inhalants suggested for catarrh (see p. 68) can often help.

If there is any discharge or possibility that the eardrum has burst then seek immediate medical help.

For minor cases, where there is no risk that the eardrum has perforated, ear drops using infused St. John's wort oil are safe to use. Put a few drops in the ear and then insert a cotton ball. Repeat 3 or 4 times a day as needed. Massaging the mastoid bone (behind the ear) with antiseptic oils can also help. Use 10 drops of lavender oil in a teaspoon of almond or vegetable oil, or 2 drops of tea tree oil applied directly. A traditional cure was to insert the heart of a freshly boiled onion into the ear—a suitably hot and ideally shaped healing poultice if nothing else is available.

Take 2 200-mg capsules of echinacea 3 times a day

to combat the infection or eat plenty of garlic at each meal.

EYE PROBLEMS

Herbal remedies can be helpful for a number of eye problems although, if symptoms persist, it is best to seek professional treatment.

Blepharitis. This is an inflammation of the eyelid often caused by an allergic reaction to cosmetics. In chronic cases the eyelid can become ulcerated with a yellow crust, the eyelashes often became matted and may fall out. Use a little marigold cream or infused marigold oil to smear gently onto the eyelid. If available, echinacea or chamomile creams can be used instead.

Conjunctivitis. Also known as pink eye, conjunctivitis is an inflammation of the fine membrane (conjunctiva) covering the eyeball. Sufferers usually complain of severe pain, watering and a "gritty feeling" on blinking. Use a decoction (1 teaspoon to 2 cups of water) of marigold, elderflower or eyebright in an eyewash (see p. 19); repeat 4 times a day. Diluted apple juice is another alternative; add 1 teaspoon of organic juice (without preservatives) to 1 tablespoon of water.

Styes: Styes are an acute inflammation of a gland at the base of an eyelash, usually caused by bacterial infection. They can indicate lowered resistance due to stress, overwork or repeated infection. Apply a little marigold, echinacea or chamomile cream directly to the stye or soak a piece of cotton cloth in marigold or elderflower infusion or distilled witch hazel; press it to the closed eye and hold it there for several minutes.

Repeat as often as possible. Internally take garlic or echinacea capsules to combat the infection; even better, learn to relax or use Siberian ginseng (p. 42) to help the body cope more effectively with stress.

Tired Eyes: Too much reading, too long at the computer screen or too much time in a smoky or polluted atmosphere—whatever the cause, tired, strained eyes are commonplace. They can be relieved by applying slices of cucumber or soaked fennel or chamomile tea bags over the closed eyes as you lie down and relax for 10 minutes. Drink the chamomile tea before using the tea bag in this way to further encourage relaxation!

FLATULENCE

Gas is usually more of an embarrassment than an indicator of serious health problems. Diet is often the problem. Some foods are essentially very "windy;" old herbals usually stress this point about beans and the cabbage family, and traditional recipes usually add carminative herbs to these foods to reduce the problem. Adding fennel, rosemary or sage to the cooking pot not only improves the flavor but also introduces herbs that stimulate and soothe the digestive system, thus reducing the risk of gas and indigestion. Similarly, cutting down on dairy, wheat, alcohol and sugary foods can be beneficial.

Drinking a carminative tea such as chamomile, peppermint, fennel or lemon balm (1 teaspoon to 1 cup of water) *after* meals is also helpful. A cup of sage tea, made in the same way, taken 3 times a day *before* meals will help to tonify a weak digestion and improve function. (See also **Indigestion,** p. 85.)

FRACTURES

Broken bones need professional treatment, although in the past, that treatment would have relied heavily on herbs. After any accident where movement of a limb is impaired or where there is severe bruising and pain, an x-ray is essential to identify cracks and fractures. Immobilize affected bones as much as possible, and head for the emergency room.

For minor cracks or breaks in toes or ribs, orthodox medicine has little to offer but firm bandages and bed rest, so additional herbal self-help is possible. Comfrey, once known as knitbone, is the herb of choice. In traditional medicine, the leaves would have been pulped into a paste which was spread onto the affected area to form a thick crust. This hardened to form a splint-like support and provided healing chemicals to be absorbed through the skin. Try to apply comfrey ointment or infused oil to the damaged tissues as soon as possible after the accident. Arnica cream can also help to relieve pain and encourage healing while taking homeopathic arnica 6x internally will also speed repair. Take 1 tablet every 15 to 30 minutes for 2 hours or until you feel less traumatized.

GASTRITIS

Gastritis simply means an inflammation of the stomach lining and is often the result of overindulgence in rich foods and alcohol. Symptoms can include nausea, vomiting and diarrhea and are very similar to food poisoning; if several members of the family or fellow dinner guests are affected then this is probably the cause (see

p. 75). Chronic gastritis increases the risk of developing stomach or duodenal ulcers and is often associated with smoking or alcoholism. Those prone to gastritis should avoid irritant foods (spices, tea, coffee, alcohol, fried foods and pickles) and eat smaller meals more regularly.

The herbal approach includes soothing mucilages and anti-inflammatories with herbs that will cover and protect the stomach lining and encourage healing. Slippery elm is ideal either taken in tablet form or as a gruel (p. 44). Licorice is also helpful; make a strong decoction by heating half a cup of chopped dried licorice root in 1 pint of water and simmer until the volume is reduced by two-thirds; then combine with 2 tablespoons of honey (which acts as a preservative) and heat to form a thin syrup. Take 1 to 2 teaspoons of the mixture up to 4 times a day. It will generally keep for up to two weeks in the refrigerator stored in a small jar. Eating a bowl of stewed apples once or twice a day can also help.

You can make a soothing tea by mixing equal amounts of chamomile flowers and meadowsweet and using 2 teaspoons to a cup of water. If available, add a teaspoon of the licorice and honey mix to each cup.

HANGOVERS

Too much alcohol not only leads to gastritis but to the headaches, dry mouth, increased urination and the muzziness of a hangover as well. The symptoms are actually those of poisoning. Drink plenty of water, diluted fruit juice, black tea or black coffee and take herbs to help cool and soothe any related stomach inflammation (such as the gastritis tea given above). This will help to flush the poisons out of the system as well as combat the symptoms of nausea. It is also important to help restore normal liver function. Evening primrose oil can be helpful; take up to 2 g in capsules on "the morning after" and add a vitamin B-complex supplement as well. Eat mashed bananas on wholemeal bread to help restore lowered potassium levels.

Although high alcohol consumption is best avoided, taking a couple of slippery elm capsules before imbibing will help lower alcohol absorption while milk thistle seeds (*Carduus marianus*) are also known to protect the liver. Take 1 teaspoon of seeds in a cup of water as an infusion or use 10 drops of commercially made tincture before a party if you intend to drink alcoholic beverages.

HAY FEVER AND ALLERGIC RHINITIS

Hay fever is usually associated with grass pollen allergies in the summer months although it can be triggered by all sorts of allergens ranging from house dust and car fumes to fungal spores in late autumn. Typical symptoms include sneezing, sore and watering eyes, a runny nose and drowsiness. Around 15 percent of teenagers tend to be affected and it is a major cause of missed exams and absenteeism. The physical symptoms are largely due to the body's production of histamine as it attempts to rid itself of the allergen.

Herbal treatment can involve strengthening the mucous membranes well before the hay fever season arrives plus remedies to provide symptomatic relief. Beginning in January or February, drink a cup of the following herbal tea each day for six weeks:

Hay Fever Prevention Tea

2 parts each ribwort plantain and elderflower
1 part each chamomile and sage

Mix the herbs and use 1 teaspoon to a cup of water.

To relieve symptoms during the hay fever season, use a tea containing equal amounts of sage and eyebright (1 teaspoon to 1 cup, up to 4 times a day) or take 2 200-mg capsules containing powdered eyebright each morning. A steam inhalation (p. 55) made from 1 tablespoon of chamomile or yarrow flowers or 10 drops of thyme oil to 1 quart of boiling water can help relieve the symptoms of nasal congestion and watery eyes.

Avoid all dairy products, coffee and alcohol during the hay fever season; try a fruit fast once a week (no food except up to 12 pieces of fruit each day) and eat a raw vegetable salad at least once a day.

In allergic rhinitis the hay fever symptoms can continue for much of the year and may be due to dust, house mites or animal hairs. Use antiallergenic bedding, mattress and pillow liners, and vacuum mattresses, upholstery and carpets at least once a day. For allergic skin rashes see p. 88.

HEADACHES AND MIGRAINES

Herbalists tend to regard headaches as symptoms of some underlying disorder rather than an illness in its own right; those that seem centered behind the eyes suggest a digestive disturbance while headaches that seem to start at the back of the neck and creep forward are generally tension headaches. Pain and sensitivity around the eyes or above the nose can be due to a sinus problem (see page 67).

Muscle strain in the shoulders and neck can also contribute to head pain. Sitting or working awkwardly hunched over a desk or computer keyboard can easily lead to headaches. Massage neck and shoulders with a mixture of 5 drops each of thyme, lavender and juniper oil in 1 tablespoon of almond oil.

Tension Tea

1 part each chamomile flowers and St. John's wort
2 parts each skullcap and lavender flowers

Mix the herbs and make an infusion using 2 teaspoons of the mix to each cup of boiling water. Drink the tea as soon as headache symptoms appear, sipping it slowly, relaxing and doing nothing else at the same time.

Take a 600-mg tablet of Siberian ginseng each day to improve stress tolerance and thus reduce the risk of tension headaches and try yoga or tai ch'i classes to improve relaxation skills.

Some sorts of headaches are best relieved by a hot towel on the head; in these cases use a massage of 10 drops of rosemary oil to 1 teaspoon of almond oil on the temples and forehead.

Migraine is typically preceded by visual disturbances: jagged lights to the edge of the visual field or a sense that there is a strange out-of-focus area in what one sees. Occasionally the attack may simply comprise these visual upsets although more usually a severe headache will follow with increased sensitivity to light so that sufferers want simply to lie down in a dark room. Migraines can be associated with gastric disturbances (nausea and vomiting) or pins and needles in one hand or arm. Foods can often trigger an attack (especially red wine, chocolate, pork, citrus fruits, coffee and cheese) or an attack can be associated with stress or bright sunlight. Flickering lights, as when driving past trees on a bright sunny day, can also trigger an attack.

Many sufferers find that chewing feverfew leaves can help prevent attacks: try 2 to 3 leaves in a daily sandwich (see p. 21 for cautions) or else use a strong lavender oil rub (1 teaspoon of lavender oil with 2 teaspoons of almond oil) massaged into the temples at the first hint of a migraine. Drink cups of lavender and St. John's wort infusion (1 teaspoon of each to a cup of water) during attacks.

For headaches associated with digestive upsets try an infusion containing 1 teaspoon each of peppermint and fennel to a cup of water.

Persistent or sudden unusually severe headaches lasting for three days or more should be referred to a medical practitioner.

INDIGESTION AND HEARTBURN

Heartburn, pain in the lower chest, flatulence and nausea are extremely common, and few sufferers ever seek professional help, preferring instead to try an assortment of antacid remedies to solve the problem. Unfortunately, trying to reduce the normal acid secretions of the stomach artificially simply encourages it to produce even more, so over-the-counter antacids can be counterproductive.

The herbal approach is to combine aromatic carminatives to ease flatulence and nausea with relaxing herbs that can reduce the anxiety and tension that often contribute to the problem. Add soothing demulcents to help protect the stomach from excess acid and perhaps a bitter to stimulate the digestive process and restore normal function.

Tea for Good Digestion

2 parts each chamomile and meadowsweet
1 part each peppermint and lemon balm

Mix the herbs and make an infusion using 2 teaspoons to a cup of water. Add a pinch of powdered nutmeg or cinnamon and drink before meals.

Slippery elm tablets or gruel taken before a meal can also help (see p. 44), especially if there is any heartburn. This is common in chronic obesity and pregnancy because the stomach is forced upwards and the diaphragm, which divides the esophagus from the stomach and normally prevents food returning to the gullet, is weakened. Acid reflux thus occurs with the highly acidic contents of the stomach returning to the esophagus, which can lead to inflammation and eventually ulceration. A hiatus hernia, in which part of the stomach is forced upwards through the diaphragm, can cause similar high acidity problems. Raising the head of the bed 6-8 inches by putting bricks under the legs will prevent acid from leaking out of the stomach and can prove a very simple way of reducing symptoms, which are generally worse at night.

Carminative teas taken with meals instead of coffee can also help; fennel, peppermint or chamomile, which are all generally available in tea bags from health food stores and restaurants, are worth trying.

If nausea is a problem, drink a tea of 1 to 2 slices of fresh ginger root simmered with 1½ cups of water in a decoction.

The pain of indigestion can sometimes be confused with heart pain from disorders like angina pectoris. Heart pain eases with rest, while heartburn is generally worse when the sufferer lies down. Sudden severe "indigestion" in someone who has previously been symptom-free should always be professionally investigated for a possible underlying heart condition. Chronic indigestion can also be a sign of peptic ulcers, gallbladder disorders, liver problems or cancer, and expert diagnosis is essential.

INSECT BITES AND STINGS

For most people, insect bites and stings lead to little more than local irritation which eases in a few days, although for an unfortunate minority certain types of stings can lead to severe allergic reactions that may be fatal. Typical symptoms include dizziness, sickness, breathing problems and marked swelling of the affected area. Immediate emergency medical treatment is vital in such cases.

Bees will only sting if they or their hives are attacked, as the hooked barb on the sting cannot be withdrawn and the insect dies defending itself. Make sure you remove any remaining sting with tweezers before cleaning and treating the wound. Wasps have a straight sting and can repeatedly attack their victims. Bee stings are acidic and, in traditional first aid, were treated with bicarbonate of soda, while alkaline wasp stings can be soothed by vinegar. Both types, however, respond well to slices of onion.

Mosquitoes and gnats can be troublesome in the summer, and in sensitive individuals, can lead to weeping sores that will take several days to heal.

Generally soothing for most types of insect bites and stings are slices of cucumber or tomato, fresh lemon juice, green tea or fresh plantain leaves. Tea tree oil, sage or lemon balm ointments are also useful standbys to keep in the first aid kit. If bites become infected or weeping, use marigold, tea tree, echinacea or St. John's wort cream or oils.

Aloe vera plants also contain a cooling sap that will reduce irritation. If you have a plant, simply split open a leaf and apply it directly to the affected area. The sap remains liquid for several hours, so keep the leaf by you and simply reapply as the irritation develops. Keeping insects away is also important; see p. 107 for some suggestions.

ITCHINESS AND SKIN RASHES

Itching skin has many causes–from contact with an obvious allergen like stinging nettles which produces the irritant weals of nettle rash (urticaria or hives) to nervous problems, certain liver disorders and drug allergies. As always, identifying the cause is important, and persistent itching for no apparent reason should be referred to a health care professional.

In most cases allergic rashes from eating certain foods such as shellfish or strawberries or contact with irritants will fade within a few hours, but in severe cases there may be swelling of the hands, face, arms, eyelids or throat with painful joints or breathing problems which can require emergency treatment.

Itching can be soothed with a lotion made by combining marigold or chamomile infusion (2 teaspoons of petals or flowers to a cup of water) with an equal amount of distilled witch hazel and applying this with a cotton swab to the affected area. Alternatively, add 2 drops of lavender or peppermint oil to a teaspoon of marigold or chickweed cream, mix well and use that instead. Borage juice (*Borago officinalis*) is also very effective in easing itching rashes or you can use aloe vera gel (as for insect bites). Fresh chickweed or plantain leaves pulped in a food processor can also be used as a lotion.

One of the most common causes of skin rashes is salicylate allergy. Salicylates are chemicals found in most fruits and vegetables (notably strawberries and tomatoes) and also form the basis of aspirin. The rash often appears around the mouth very soon after eating salicylate-rich foods and can be persistent. The condition often seems to develop in the elderly who have been told to take daily doses of aspirin in an attempt to counter the risk of heart disorders. A low-salicylate diet is important (lists of high-salicylate foods are available in many popular books on nutrition) as is avoiding salicylate-containing drugs.

Other drugs, including some antibiotics, can have a similar effect, so always check with your practitioner if skin rashes follow a new prescription.

Contact irritants are equally numerous; insect stings, especially bee stings and bee products, cosmetics, perfumes and a large number of common garden plants can cause urticaria.

JOINT PAIN AND STIFFNESS

Arthritis, one of the most common causes of joint pain and stiffness, is not really a "first aid" problem since the condition tends to be chronic, persistent and long-term. It is generally treated internally using anti-inflammatories (see *Herbs to Relieve Arthritis* by CJ Puotinen, Keats, 1996) although emergency short-term relief for osteoarthritis can be achieved by using rosemary oil externally. Mix 1 teaspoon of rosemary oil with 1 tablespoon of almond oil and massage into aching joints. Eating a daily bowl of cucumber soup can also help in the long term.

For joints that feel hot and swollen, use an ice pack (or package of frozen peas) to cool the affected area and then massage gently with a mixture of 1 teaspoon of infused St. John's wort oil with 20 drops of essential oil of lavender.

General stiffness, following gardening or sports, can be helped by a hot bath to which 5 drops each of rosemary, thyme, and juniper essential oils have been added. Use strained infusions (2 teaspoons to a cup of water) of rosemary and thyme if you don't have the essential oils. Local stiffness can also be helped by a cabbage leaf poultice; simply soften the leaf with a vegetable mallet and hold in place with a loose bandage.

Internally, meadowsweet and St. John's wort tea (1 teaspoon of each to a cup of water) can help to relieve pain in the short term, although if the condition persists for more than 48 hours or worsens, seek professional help.

MENSTRUAL PROBLEMS

Herbal medicine can be extremely effective for treating menstrual disorders. As always, identifying the underlying cause of the problem is vital for accurate treatment.

Heavy menstrual flow. Persistent problems should be referred to a specialist for accurate diagnosis, but an occasional excessive flow can be helped with stinging nettle and yarrow tea (1 teaspoon of each to 1 cup of water). Persistent heavy menstrual blood loss can lead to anemia so add iron-rich foods like liver, apricots, watercress and parsley to the diet or take supplements of Dong Quai (*Angelica polymorpha* var. *sinensis*) available from health food stores.

Menstrual pain. Try St. John's wort tea and raspberry leaf (*Rubus idaeus*) tea (1 teaspoon of each to a cup of water), marigold infusion (p. 31) or massage 5 drops of sage oil in 1 teaspoon of almond oil over the lower abdomen. If available, 2 teaspoons of black haw tincture (*Viburnum prunifolium*) in half a glass of hot water will often bring rapid and lasting relief. Exercise often helps, so rather than curling up with a hot water bottle and feeling miserable, take a brisk walk. Regular sexual intercourse in the days before a period can also reduce the likelihood of painful menstruation.

Vaginal itching. This is often related to fungal infections (see p. 101) and can be associated with recurrent bouts of cystitis. It is also common in post-menopausal women. Marigold, tea tree and vitamin E creams can all bring relief. If it is available, add 1 drop of rose oil (*Rosa damascena*) to 1 teaspoon of marigold cream: mix well and use night and morning.

MOUTH ULCERS

Mouth ulcers (or aphtha) are commonly occurring lesions found on the tongue, roof of the mouth and inside the cheeks. They usually start with a red, sore patch of blisters erupting to produce a greyish white ulcer. They can occur singly or in groups and will usually clear of their own accord after a week or so but can be so painful that eating becomes almost impossible.

They often erupt when the sufferer is tired, over-stressed or fighting an infection and may be associated with digestive disorders and stomach upsets. Mouth ulcers are generally more common in those suffering from yeast infections or candidiasis. If mouth ulcers are a recurrent problem, try immune-stimulant tonics; eat plenty of garlic and shiitake mushrooms or take a course of Korean ginseng (*Panax ginseng*) tablets (600 mg a day for 1 month).

Herbal mouth washes can bring symptomatic relief; try using sage or rosemary infusion (1 teaspoon to a cup of water, strained, and use to thoroughly rinse the mouth 3-4 times a day). Alternatively, add 20 drops of clove oil to half a glass of warm water and use that instead.

MUSCULAR PAINS, STRAINS AND SPRAINS

Pulled muscles and twisted joints can be acutely painful and, if caused by some traumatic injury, an x-ray is advisable to identify fractures. Strains involve a slight tearing of a muscle or the tendon attaching it to a bone and are generally caused by overstretching. Sprains are a tear in the joint capsule or associated ligaments caused by twisting. Muscular aches and pains can also be associated with rheumatism and inflammation of the muscle or associated soft tissues.

Comfrey or arnica used externally is an ideal first aid remedy to help repair damaged tissues. Arnica can be particularly useful for relieving pain while comfrey actually increases cell growth and so speeds healing. Do not use either ointment if the skin is broken.

Twisted or strained muscles will also respond well to herbal massage rubs. Combine 5 drops each of thyme, rosemary, and lavender essential oils with 1 teaspoon of almond oil and massage gently into affected areas.

For rheumatic pains, combine the external massage oils with 2 to 3 daily cups of meadowsweet tea (1 teaspoon of herb per cup). Oatstraw baths are also worth trying (p. 34).

NAUSEA AND VOMITING

Nausea and vomiting can be associated with a wide range of illnesses: from life-threatening fevers and stomach problems to motion sickness, migraines and indigestion. It is important to seek professional help for severe and persistent problems, but minor disorders, with a clear cause, can be helped by herbal remedies at home. Caution is needed, however, as many herbs are quite unpleasant to taste, and for sufferers who dislike the flavor they can increase rather than ease symptoms.

For nausea associated with stomach upsets, lemon balm or chamomile can be helpful. Drink 1 cup of tea (containing 1 teaspoon of herb) every 2 to 3 hours until symptoms ease.

Ginger is one of the most effective antiemetics in the repertoire and can be taken in the form of ginger wine, ginger ale or ginger snaps if the actual herb is not available. Otherwise make a decoction of ginger (simmer 1 to 2 slices of fresh root in 1½ cups of water) and sip that. You can boil the decoction down to 1 to 2 tablespoons and take in drop doses if that is easier to swallow.

Ginger is quite safe to take for morning sickness during pregnancy and has been prescribed in doses of up to 1 g at a time in clinical trials with no ill effects.[4] A useful way to take remedies at this time is to fill a thermos bottle with an infusion of either fennel, lemon balm, chamomile or peppermint (using 1 tablespoon of herb to a quart of water) and leave by the bedside table so that the tea can be sipped before arising. For those who dislike herbal teas, use 5 to 10 drops of commercially made tincture either placed directly on the tongue or diluted in a little warm water. If possible give yourself a choice of morning teas each day as, depending on mood, some may prove more effective than others.

NEURALGIA

Neuralgia simply means nerve pain and usually involves an inflammation of the nerve fibers. It can occur anywhere but most commonly affects the trigeminal nerve which runs along the side of the face and scalp. It is often exacerbated by cold and drafts. A little lemon juice or a slice of lemon applied to the area can help; warm the lemon slightly under a grill rather than using directly from the refrigerator.

Alternatively, use 5 drops of lavender essential oil in a teaspoon of either St. John's wort infused oil or cayenne infused oil (p. 56) and dab gently onto the affected area. Internally, a cup of tea containing 1 teaspoon each of St. John's wort and skullcap can be helpful. Eating cooked oatmeal for breakfast each morning will also provide a good restoring tonic for the nervous system.

NOSEBLEEDS

Persistent nosebleeds can suggest elevated blood pressure or other disorders and should be professionally investigated. The sort which accompany colds or traumatic injury can be quickly stopped by inserting a freshly gathered yarrow leaf in the nostril. If that is not available, then insert a cotton ball soaked in distilled witch hazel, lemon juice or marigold infusion instead and drink the remainder of the cup of marigold tea, which will also help. Pinching the nostrils together and leaning forward will quickly stop a minor nosebleed. If it is associated with catarrh or a cold, then drink up to 3 cups a day of eyebright or elderflower infusion (1 teaspoon to a cup of water).

SHOCK

Calming herbs are ideal for any sort of shock; use 2 teaspoons of skullcap, lemon balm or chamomile to a cup of water and sip slowly. Homeopathic arnica 6x is ideal if the shock follows some sort of accident, such as a fall, and will help speed tissue repair as well.

Bach Flower Rescue Remedy is also extremely helpful. Flower remedies were developed by Dr. Edward Bach in the 1930s and are made from the dew collected from flowers and preserved with a little brandy. Rescue Remedy is a combination of cherry plum, which Dr. Bach believed was good for loss of control, clematis for unconsciousness, impatiens for stress, rock rose for terror and star of Bethlehem for shock. Add 2 to 3 drops of Rescue Remedy to a cup of calming tea (such as skullcap or chamomile) or put 1 to 2 drops directly onto the tongue.

Rescue Remedy is also available as a cream which can be massaged into the temples if the sufferer is unconscious, and is well worth keeping in the first aid kit for emergencies.

SLEEPLESSNESS

The amount of sleep we each need varies and at some times we need more sleep than at others. A couple of bad nights are generally followed by a night of good deep sleep and the body usually "catches up" on lost sleep over a few days. Sleeplessness becomes a problem when sufferers feel tired and unable to concentrate during the day or when it becomes a worry in itself with seemingly endless hours spent tossing and turning in bed at night.

There are many causes for disturbed sleep patterns. Heavy meals late at night can lead to disturbed digestion; painful joints and muscles or irritating coughs will keep most people awake; and catnapping during the day simply fills up the sleep quota and there is no need for further rest. Commonly, insomnia is associated with tension and worries and a failure to relax before bedtime. Sedative and relaxing herbs to help reduce anxieties and calm an overactive mind will often encourage sleep. They are also non-addictive, although some find that with regular use the potency of herbal insomnia remedies is reduced and it can be worthwhile changing the mix regularly if long-term use is likely.

If relaxation is a problem, try a hot soak in the tub before bed adding 1 to 2 drops of lavender or chamomile oil, or 2 cups of strained infusion (2 teaspoons of herb per cup) of either herb, to the bath water. Follow the bath with a cup of tea containing 1 teaspoon each of St. John's wort and chamomile and head for bed.

For small children 1 to 3 cups of chamomile tea in the bath water will often calm the most restless toddler; alternatively, put one drop of chamomile oil on nightwear or the pillow.

Other herbs which can be especially good for insomnia are passionflower (*Passiflora incarnata*) and Californian poppy (*Eschscholzia Californica*), which are both available as tablets or tinctures and can be grown in most gardens. Use the aerial parts in each case and make a tea containing 1 to 2 teaspoons of herb to a cup. A pillow stuffed with fresh hops (*Humulus lupulus*) is another traditional and very effective remedy for insomnia. A pleasant-tasting combination for restful sleep follows.

Sleep Tea

2 parts each passionflower and California poppy
1 part each St. John's wort, skullcap and lavender

Mix the herbs and make an infusion using 2 teaspoons to a cup of boiling water. Drink 30 minutes before bedtime.

SORE THROAT AND LARYNGITIS

For many people a sore throat can be the first sign of a developing cold or it could herald laryngitis (inflammation of the voice box or larynx and vocal cords), tonsillitis or German measles. The inflammation may be caused by viral or bacterial infection, and recurrence can be associated with stress or a reduced resistance to infection. With laryngitis there is generally hoarseness or even a complete loss of voice.

The tonsils are small packs of lymphatic tissue at the back of the throat which help protect the body from infection. Recurrent tonsillitis can often indicate some underlying stress on the system, such as food allergy, with the immune system having to work overtime to combat the problem. In severe cases the tonsils can become filled with pus, causing an abscess which can need surgical treatment.

Mild sore throats will often clear in two or three days with or without treatment, but if symptoms persist for more than a few days, then professional investigation is needed in case there is some major problem, such as a growth, causing the hoarseness.

Gargles of any astringent herb will generally be helpful—try sage, rosemary, marigold or fennel using 2 teaspoons of herb to a cup of boiling water in each case. Allow the mixture to cool thoroughly before straining and using as a gargle. Adding a small pinch of cayenne powder can be helpful, but do not put in too much as it makes the gargle very warming indeed. Also effective is gargling with either diluted lemon juice or fresh pineapple juice. Tinctures can be used instead of infusions: add 1 teaspoon of echinacea or sage tincture to ½ cup of warm water. If the tonsils are infected, gargle with an infusion containing 1 teaspoon each of thyme, sage and elderflower to a cup of water and take 3 200-mg capsules of echinacea up to 3 times a day.

Sore throats also need soothing foods and drinks; eat 1 to 2 teaspoons of honey mixed in a serving of ice cream or drink the juice of a lemon in a cup of hot water with 2 teaspoons of honey added.

SPLINTERS

Most splinters can be easily removed with the help of a sterilized needle and tweezers with a little marigold or tea tree cream then applied to the area as an antiseptic. Splinters which are difficult to dislodge can be helped by drawing ointments: apply either commercially available chickweed or slippery elm ointment and cover with a Band-Aid overnight. This will generally help dislodge deep-seated splinters which can then be removed with tweezers. Use 1 teaspoon of slippery elm powder made into a paste with a very little water as an alternative if you do not have a suitable ointment.

STOMACH UPSETS

Minor stomach upsets, with abdominal pain, nausea, diarrhea and vomiting are commonplace and can be associated with food poisoning (see p. 75), an excess of rich food or too much alcohol leading to gastritis (see p. 80). Other stomach upsets are linked to chills. When warming herbs can be useful, try the following tea:

Warming Tea

1 slice fresh ginger root
1 teaspoon lemon balm

Simmer the ginger in 1½ cups of water for 20

minutes and then pour the liquid over the lemon balm and infuse for a further 10 minutes. Strain and drink up to 3 cups daily.

Some people are rather more prone to stomach upsets than others, and the problem can be stress-related with any increase in nervous tension or anxiety levels leading to stomach discomfort. Relaxing herbs such as lemon balm and chamomile teas can be useful in these cases (use 2 teaspoons of herb to 1 cup of water and drink up to 3 times daily).

TENNIS ELBOW

Tennis elbow is a painful inflammation of the tendon at the outer edge of the elbow usually caused by excessive exercise—hence the name. As this is an inflammatory problem, direct application of herbal anti-inflammatories can often help. Add 5 drops each of lavender oil and either yarrow or chamomile oil to 1 teaspoon of St. John's wort oil and massage into the area 3 to 4 times daily.

TOOTHACHE AND GUM PROBLEMS

An an emergency remedy while awaiting dental treatment, cloves are the ideal choice for toothache. Put 2 to 3 drops of clove oil on the gum next to the tooth or suck a dried clove, holding the flower bud as close as possible to the painful tooth. You can put the oil on a cotton swab and hold it against the gum if you prefer.

Peppermint oil can be used in the same way, although it is not quite so effective.

If a filling has come out, then make a firm paste from slippery elm powder and water and put that in the hole until a dentist can fill the cavity properly. After extractions, take arnica 6x tablets 2 to 3 times daily for 2 to 3 days and use a mouth rinse made from sage infusion (1 teaspoon of herb to a cup of boiling water) with a pinch of salt as often as possible.

Bleeding gums can be eased by mouth washes of sage, marigold or eyebright infusion; use 2 teaspoons to a cup of water and rinse the mouth thoroughly every 2 to 3 hours. Add a pinch of salt to the mixture to increase the antiseptic effect.

Persistent gum problems need professional help as they may eventually cause teeth to loosen and fall out.

VAGINAL YEAST INFECTIONS

This fungal infection, characterized by a milky discharge and itching that commonly occurs in the vagina, is often associated with excessive use of antibiotics (which can damage the body's own beneficial bacteria) and also with the spermicides used in contraception. Try to restore the bacterial balance by taking 2 to 4 capsules of *Lactobacillus acidophilus*—a friendly bacteria which inhabits our digestive tracts—or eat 2 to 3 servings of plain yoghurt with active cultures daily. Avoid sugar, fermented foods or alcohol, which all encourage yeasts.

Drink up to 3 cups of marigold tea (2 teaspoons to each cup) during the day and use at least 2 cloves of garlic in cooking as well. Echinacea decoction (1 teaspoon of root per cup) can be used instead of marigold.

Topical vaginal treatment is possible using 2 to 3 drops of tea tree oil on a tampon. Simply push about ¼ inch of the tampon out of the applicator and moisten with 3 drops of tea tree oil in ½ teaspoon water. Push the tampon back, insert into the vagina and leave it there for no more than 3 hours. Repeat 2 to 3 times a day.

Marigold or tea tree cream can be used directly in the vagina instead or use tea tree pessaries, available from health stores.

WARTS

Warts are benign lumps in the skin caused by a virus which makes the cells multiply abnormally quickly. Common warts are usually found on the hands, knees and face and are mildly contagious, spreading as the virus comes into contact with damaged skin or when flakes from the wart touch nearby moist skin areas. Although they can be unsightly and a nuisance, these sorts of warts are usually quite harmless and most will disappear of their own accord—eventually. Like many common viruses, the one causing warts can remain dormant, reappearing from time to time. Warts are most common in younger people.

There is, of course, a wealth of folkloric tradition surrounding warts—they could be charmed, "sold," tied off with horse's hair, or rubbed with bacon fat which was then nailed to a door post and, as it rotted, it was believed the wart would disappear. A more practical herbal alternative is to put 1 drop of tea tree oil onto the wart night and morning. You can also squeeze 1 to 2 drops of dandelion (*Taraxacum officinale*) sap or the bright yellow sap of greater celandine (*Chelidonium major*) directly onto the wart each day if you have access to these fresh plants.

Plantar warts occur on the soles of the feet. Because they are always being walked on, the small growths can become painful and are often covered by thickened areas of skin or calluses. The constant pressure also makes these warts grow inward rather than erupting outwards as with common warts. Persistent cases usually need treatment from a chiropodist. For mild cases, tea tree cream used 2 to 3 times a day can be helpful.

Venereal or genital warts are found around the genitals and anus. They will usually disappear of their own accord, but because of the contagious nature of viruses they can be transmitted during sexual intercourse. These warts need professional treatment. Professional help is also needed for warts which erupt at the site of moles or which start to bleed or change color.

First Aid For Travelers

Travel—be it to some exotic location or simply to a neighboring state—can bring its own health hazards. Jet lag, stomach upsets from unfamiliar foods, sunburn and travel sickness are all too familiar to the traveler. Packing a few essential herbal remedies before you head for the airport can save hours of wasted vacation time searching for pharmacists or seeking professional medical help for minor ills.

In less developed countries it is best to avoid eating any raw foods and drinking tap water to reduce the risk of gastric upsets. In hot climates, too much fruit is not a good idea either—especially if you are coming from cooler zones. In Chinese terms, most fruit is characterized as *yin* and is very cooling. Those arriving in the tropics from temperate areas are already sufficiently *"yin"* in character so adding more fruit to the system can result in ailments associated with over-chilled stomachs, including diarrhea and abdominal bloating. Wait for a few days to become acclimatized to the new temperatures before gorging on guavas, mangoes or other exotica. If stomach upsets strike before then, switch to eating papaya (*Carica papaya*)—a traditional and effective remedy for stomach ills used throughout the Far East.

Fortunately, if you are traveling in Europe, even

if you forget to pack essential herbs, they will probably be available in local health food stores and pharmacies. Homeopathic remedies are readily available in European pharmacies and the botanical Latin names for tinctures or dried herbs will be the same in any language.

To be on the safe side, choose your essentials for your travel first aid kit from the remedies and self-help suggestions below (botanical names are given for those plants not included in Chapter 2).

CUTS AND SCRAPES (see p. 74)

- Pack a small bottle containing equal amounts of St. John's wort and marigold tinctures and use 1 teaspoon to a cup of boiled water to bathe cuts and scrapes. Press a clean handkerchief to the cut to help stop bleeding and apply a Band-Aid if needed.
- A small bottle of distilled witch hazel can be used instead and will also be helpful to soothe sunburn, sprains and bruises.

DIARRHEA AND STOMACH UPSETS

These are all-too-common problems for travelers who may find that local standards of hygiene in exotic locations are not quite the same as back home. When traveling in high risk areas never eat raw salads; always wash and peel fruit; avoid ice cubes in drinks; and regard street vendors selling "bottled water" with some suspicion. In high-risk areas, brush your teeth using bottled water or—even better—freshly made green tea.

- Pack a small bottle of meadowsweet tincture and take 10 to 20 drops in boiled water every 2 to 3 hours at the first sign of stomach upsets, gastritis or heartburn.
- Eat a raw, peeled, grated apple every 2 to 3 hours to help control diarrhea or drink a cup of strong, cold back tea without milk or sugar every 2 to 3 hours to help alleviate symptoms.
- Take a bottle containing equal amount of tinctures of agrimony (*Agrimonia eupatoria*) and gotu kola (*Centella asiatica*) in your luggage and take 2 teaspoons in ½ cup of boiled or bottled water every 3 hours for the more troublesome sorts of travel diarrhea.

HEAT STROKE

Symptoms can include headache, nausea, inability to concentrate, raised temperature without sweating and a general feeling of being unwell. Heat stroke can be fatal in severe cases so do not delay in seeking medical help. Always wear a hat in hot climates, avoid lengthy exposure to the sun, and drink plenty of fluids (at least 2 quarts a day).

- Mix 1 teaspoon each of salt and sugar in a cup of water and drink every 20 to 30 minutes until symptoms ease. Bathe the forehead with lavender oil in cold water if available or soak cloths in cold water and apply to all parts of the body.

INSECT REPELLENTS, STINGS AND BITES
(see p. 87)

Insect bites can lead to all sorts of unpleasant conditions—especially as you get closer to the tropics—so the sensible thing is to avoid being bitten in the first place. Long socks can prevent sand fleas and mosquitoes from gaining hold; tuck trousers into socks when walking in sandy areas. Combine protective clothing with a light covering of an herbal insect repellent (see below). Alternatively, use the same mixture undiluted in pomander beads or decorative miniature scent bottles on a necklace to keep a slight whiff of oil around you to ward off bugs.

- Lemongrass oil (*Cymbopogon citratus*) is ideal to repel insects and avoid those troublesome bites that can spoil a trip. Dilute the oil to no more than 5 percent concentration (20 drops in a tablespoon of almond oil) and cover areas of exposed skin. A plastic spray bottle can be used for brief periods instead but will tend to clog up with prolonged use; instead use a small hand spray containing 20 drops of oil in 1 cup of water and spray all exposed areas of skin 2 to 3 times a day.
- Lemon balm, tea tree and lavender oils are almost as effective as lemongrass at helping to deter insects; use in the same way.
- For insect bites, use the same mixture of St. John's wort and marigold tinctures suggested for cuts and scrapes and dilute 1 teaspoon in a cup of water to bathe affected areas as required. Look for plantain leaves locally and apply them fresh.
- Take a jar of tea tree, sage or lemon balm cream in your travel kit and apply any of these frequently to soothe insect bites.

JET LAG

It can take time for the body clock to adjust to the changes of transcontinental travel while long flights can be extremely dehydrating and exhausting as well. Avoid alcohol and fatty foods on the day before you travel and wear loose clothing and shoes, as feet and legs will swell on long flights. Flex leg muscles or try and walk around at regular intervals during the journey and take an inflatable neck pillow for extra comfort. Remember to set your watch to the time at your destination as soon as you get into the departure lounge and behave as if that were the time. Jet lag is as much a mental as a physical adaption problem.

- Take 2 200-mg capsules of Siberian ginseng each morning for 3 days before you travel and 2 days afterward. Repeat for the homeward journey.
- Use chamomile or lime flower (*Tilia europaea*) tea in flight instead of coffee or alcohol and save the tea bags to use as eye pads to relieve the irritation caused by the dry atmosphere on board the aircraft. Drink plenty of water to avoid dehydration.

SHOCK AND ACCIDENTS (see p. 95)

Don't forget to include a bottle of homeopathic arnica 6x tablets in your travel kit and take 1 to 2 at 30-minute intervals for up to 4 hours after the shock or accident or until you feel calmer.

SPRAINS AND BRUISES (see p. 92)

- Pack a tube of arnica or comfrey cream and apply as directed (neither of these creams should be used on broken skin).
- Sprains can be eased by alternately soaking the affected area in hot and iced water: 2 to 3 minutes of each for as long as you can or until bruises have fully developed.

SUNBURN

Use a high sun-protection-factor sunscreen and replace it after each vacation as it soon deteriorates. Select sunglasses with an approved sun-protection-factor label; poor quality sunglasses can do more harm than good. Wear a hat with a large brim.

- Pack a small bottle of lavender oil in infused St. John's wort oil (40 drops of lavender oil to 2 tablespoons of the St. John's wort oil) and use this as a soothing lotion for sunburned skin.
- Take a tube of aloe vera cream and use on sunburn; it will also be helpful for insect bites and minor cuts.

TRAVEL SICKNESS

Whether it occurs in trains, planes, boats or cars, travel sickness soon becomes a problem for the entire family. Symptoms start with pallor, sweating and nausea and soon lead to vomiting and faintness and can be brought on by general stuffiness and lack of fresh air, mild claustrophobia, and the all-pervading smell of diesel and engine oil still occasionally encountered on ferries.

Children's ears tend to be more sensitive to motion disturbances, and travel sickness is thus more commonplace among the young and is often something they outgrow.

- Ginger in any form is ideal; take 1 to 2 200-mg capsules or 10 drops of diluted tincture before traveling. Dilute a teaspoon of tincture in a tablespoon of water and store this in a dropper bottle; add comforting drops to the tongue if a sea-crossing becomes extra choppy or the car journey becomes jerky.
- For young children who cannot swallow capsules, use any ginger-based product they will tolerate— ginger ale, ginger snaps, or candied ginger sweets.
- 2 slippery elm tablets 1 to 2 hours before traveling will also help prevent nausea and vomiting.
- Drink chamomile tea on sea or air voyages and avoid fatty foods. Bitter oranges are also ideal for reducing symptoms of motion sickness; eat marmalade at breakfast or suck orange-flavored sweets.
- Homeopathic nux vomica 6x (*Strychnos nux-vomica*) is also convenient to take for any sort of nausea and is available in easy-to-use tablets which can be put under the tongue every 1 to 2 hours as required.

HELPFUL TEA BAGS TO BRING WITH YOU

There is usually room in the suitcase for a few tea bags of single herbs for emergency use. Remember to pack:

- Fennel for indigestion and griping pains
- Chamomile for insomnia and the stress of jet lag
- Peppermint for indigestion
- Ordinary Indian tea for diarrhea
- Elderflower, both to drink for catarrh and to use dampened, as eye pads for sore, tired or irritated eyes

When To Summon Help

Most of the ills which befall us are minor, self-limiting and everyday ailments that will respond well to simple herbal remedies at home. That said, one must always be prepared for the unexpected and for those serious conditions which appear to start much as any other cold, stomach pain or headache. Self-medication always carries the risk of delay in seeking professional and relevant help. If in any doubt at all about the nature of a health problem, go to a health professional.

This is especially true if symptoms appear to be worsening; in particular do not hesitate to seek advice from doctors, nurses or hospital emergency rooms in cases when:

- Accidental falls may have resulted in a broken bone
- Abdominal pain is severe, there is excessive tenderness when the area is touched or it is associated with persistent vomiting
- There is noticeable behavioral change in babies and toddlers, especially in feeding, sleep or play
- There has been a severe blow to the head and the sufferer complains of any nausea or vomiting
- There is any major difficulty in breathing or the patient complains of chest pains
- Feverishness is accompanied by severe head pains, joint or neck stiffness, or transient rashes

- Fevers rise to more than 102°F/39°C
- There is any constant head pain for more than a few hours and the sufferer does not have a history of similar attacks or migraines
- Nosebleeds continue for more than 10 to 20 minutes or are particularly severe

Although herbal medicine is generally quite safe, it can occasionally conflict with orthodox treatments. Note the cautions listed under specific herbs, and if you are on any long-term medication seek advice from your medical practitioner or professional herbalist before taking herbs for any length of time. First-aid use in the vast majority of cases will cause no problems at all, but if you plan to take herbs for longer than a couple of days, it is best to check.

Any medication involves a degree of toxicity—a fact of which medieval herbalists were well aware. One must always treat herbs—and indeed therapeutic foods—with respect; they are potent medicines. As the great 16th century herbalist Paracelsus put it: "In all things there is poison, and there is nothing without a poison. It depends only upon the dose whether a poison is a poison or not. . . ."

Appendix

REFERENCES

1. J. M. Betz, R. M. Eppley, W. C. Taylor and D. Andrzejewski (1994). "Determination of pyrrolizidine alkaloids in commercial comfrey products" in *Journal of Pharmaceutical Sciences*, Vol. 83, No 5, pp. 649–653.
2. R. Bauer (1996). Paper presented at the symposium "Modern Treatments and Traditional Remedies," organized by the Royal Pharmaceutical Society, London, 5 July 1996.
3. D. Melchart, K. Linde, F. Worku, R. Bauer, and H. Wagner (1994). "Immunomodulation with echinacea—A systematic review of controlled clinical trials" in *Phytomedicine*, Vol. 1, pp. 245–254.
4. S. Fulder and M. Tenne (1996). "Ginger and pregnancy" in *Herbalgram*, No 38, pp. 47–51.

GLOSSARY

Allergen. Any substance which triggers an allergic response.

Alterative. A substance which improves the function of various organs—notably those involved with the breakdown and excretion of waste products—to bring about a gradual change of state.

Analgesic. Relieves pain.

Anesthetic. Causes local or general loss of sensation.

Anodyne. Allays pain.

Antibiotic. Destroys or inhibits the growth of micro-organisms such as bacteria and fungi.

Antibacterial. Destroys or inhibits the growth of bacteria.

Anti-emetic. Combats nausea.

Antifungal. Destroys or inhibits the growth of fungi.

Anthelmintic. An antiparasitic herb used to destroy intestinal worms or expel them from the body.

Anti-inflammatory. Reduces inflammation.

Antimicrobial. Destroys or inhibits the growth of micro-organisms such as bacteria and fungi.

Antirheumatic. Relieves the symptoms of rheumatism.

Antiseptic. Controls or prevents infection.

Antispasmodic. Reduces muscle spasm and tension.

Antitussive. Inhibits the cough reflex, helping to stop coughing.

Aperient. A very mild laxative.

Aphrodisiac. Promotes sexual excitement.

Astringent. Precipitates proteins from the surface of cells or membranes causing tissues to contract and tighten; forms a protective coating and stops bleeding and discharges.

Bach Flower Remedies. Extracts of flowers collected as dew and preserved in brandy, developed by Dr. Edward Bach in the 1930s and widely used to treat emotional upsets and disturbances.

Bitter. Stimulates secretion of digestive juices.

Carminative. Expels gas from the stomach and intestines to relieve flatulence, digestive colic and gastric discomfort.

Cathartic. A strong, purging laxative.

Cholagogue. Stimulates bile flow from the gallbladder and bile ducts into the duodenum.

Choleretic. Increases the secretion of bile by the liver.

Circulatory stimulant. Increases blood flow.

Cleansing herb. An herb that improves the excretion of waste products from the body.

Cooling. Used to describe herbs that are often bitter or relaxing and will help to reduce internal heat and hyperactivity.

Decongestant. Relieves congestion, usually nasal.

Demulcent. Softens and soothes damaged or inflamed surfaces, such as the gastric mucous membranes.

Diaphoretic. Increases sweating.

Diuretic. Encourages urine flow.

Emetic. Causes vomiting.

Emmenagogue. Uterine stimulant which will encourage menstrual flow; excess may lead to miscarriage in pregnancy.

Essential oils. Volatile chemicals extracted from plants by such techniques as steam distillation; highly active and aromatic.

Expectorant. Enhances the secretion of sputum from the respiratory tract so that it is easier to cough up.

Febrifuge. Reduces fever.

Flavonoids. Active plant constituents which improve the circulation and may also have diuretic, anti-inflammatory and antispasmodic effects.

Laxative. Encourages bowel motions.

Mucilage. Complex sugar molecules found in plants that are soft and slippery and provide protection for the mucous membranes and inflamed surfaces.

Nervine. Affects the nervous system; may be stimulating or sedating.

Peristalsis. The waves of involuntary contractions in the digestive tract which move food and waste products through the system.

Purgative. Drastic laxative.

Pyrrolizidine alkaloids. Chemicals found in a number of plants (including comfrey, borage, and coltsfoot) which in excess can be associated with liver damage although many regard the research evidence for this as inconclusive.

Relaxant. Relaxes tense and overactive nerves and tissues.

Rubefacient. A substance which stimulates blood flow to the skin causing local reddening.

Sedative. Reduces anxiety and tension.

Stimulant. Increases activity.

Styptic. Stops external bleeding.

Systemic. Affecting the whole body.

Tonic. Restoring, nourishing and supporting for the entire body.

Vulnerary. Wound herb.

Warming. A remedy which increases body temperature and encourages digestive function and circulation. Warming herbs are often spicy and pungent to taste.

HERB SUPPLIERS

Bay Laurel Farm, West Garzas Road, Carmel Valley, CA 93924.
Tel: (408) 659–2913.
Frontier Herbs, Box 299, Norway, Iowa 52318.
Tel: (800) 669–3275.
Herbs Products Co., 11012 Magnolia Blvd., North Hollywood,
CA 91601. Tel: (818) 984–3141.
Sage Mountain Herbs, P.O. Box 420, East Barre, VT 05649. Tel:
(802) 479–9825.

BIBLIOGRAPHY

Brown, D. (1995). *Encyclopedia of Herbs and their Uses,* Dorling Kindersley, New York.

Chevallier, A. (1996). *Encyclopedia of Medicinal Plants,* Dorling Kindersley, New York.

Foster, S., and Yue, C. (1992). *Herbal Emissaries,* Healing Arts Press, Rochester, VT.

Frawley, D., and Lad, V. (1986). *The Yoga of Herbs,* Lotus Press, Santa Fe, NM.

Hobbs, C. (1995). *Medicinal Mushrooms,* Botanica Press, Santa Cruz, CA.

Ody, P. (1993). *Complete Medicinal Herbal,* Dorling Kindersley, New York.

Ody, P. (1995). *Home Herbal,* Dorling Kindersley, New York.

Tierra, M. (1988). *Planetary Herbology,* Lotus Press, Sante Fe, NM.

Vogel, V.J. (1970). *American Indian Medicine,* University of Oklahoma Press.

Weed, S. (1986). *Wise Woman Herbal for the Childbearing Year,* Ash Tree Publishing, Woodstock, New York.

INDEX